Tarascon Publishing

T[...] cketbook

See page 208 for ordering information, or go to our website at: www.tarascon.com

AHA	Am Heart Assoc	h	hour	meq	milliequiv	PR	by rectum
bid	twice per day	Hb	hemoglobin	min	minute	prn	as needed
BP	blood pressure	HR	heart rate	ml	milliliters	qd	every day
cm	centimeters	ICP	intracranial	mo	month	qid	4 times/day
CNS	central nervous sys		pressure	NS	0.9%saline	SC	subcutaneous
CSF	cerebrospinal fluid	IM	intramuscular	O_2	oxygen	SD	standard
d	day	IO	intraosseous	OD	overdose		deviation
D_5W	5% dextrose in H_2O	IV	intravenous	PMN	neutrophil	SL	sublingual
ET	endotracheal	J	joules	PO	by mouth	tid	3 times/day
F	French	kg	kilograms	PPV	+pressure	µg	micrograms
g	grams	m^2	square meters		ventilation	yo	years old

Tarascon Adult Emergency Medicine Pocketbook, 3rd edition

ISBN 1-882742-37-0.Copyright © 2005 Mako Publishing, Winter Park, Florida. Printed in the USA. All rights reserved. Published and marketed under exclusive license by Tarascon Publishing, a division of Tarascon Inc, Lompoc, California. No portion of this publication may be reproduced or stored in a retrieval system in any form or by any means (including electronic, mechanical, photocopying, etc.) without prior written permission. The cover is a detail "Wound Man" depicting injuries from various weapons, by Parcelsus, 1536.   C6

EDITORS[1]

Steven G. Rothrock MD
Professor, Emergency
Medicine University of Florida,
Associate Professor Clinical
Sciences, Florida State Univ.,
Orlando Regional Med Ctr., FL

Steven M. Green MD
Professor Emergency Medicine
& Pediatrics, Loma Linda Univ
School of Medicine

Stephen Colucciello MD
Vice Chair, Carolinas Medical
Center, Charlotte, NC

Stephen Leech MD
Christiana Care Health
System, Newark, DE

Angela McQueen Pharm D
Partner's Community
Healthcare, Inc. Boston, MA

Joseph Pagane MD
Assist Professor EM, , Orlando
Regional Medical Center,
Orlando, FL

Sal Silvestri MD
EMS Medical Director, Orange
County, Florida, Associate
Professor Emergency
Medicine, University of Florida

[1]Work-affiliation is included for identification purposes only. The views expressed in the book do not necessarily represent the views of any listed agency, school, or hospital.

Adult Basic Resuscitation
(Perform until Advanced Resuscitation Available)

No Movement or Response

↓

Call 911 or Code Blue (if Health Care Facility) AND Obtain defibrillator (e.g. AED[1])

↓

Open **Airway** and check **Breathing**

↓

If not breathing, administer **2 Breaths** – each over 1 second with enough volume to cause chest rise

↓

Check Pulse for 10 seconds	→*Definite Pulse*→	• Administer **1 breath** every 5 to 6 seconds • Recheck pulse q 2 min

↓ *No Pulse*

• Give **30 Compressions & 2 Breaths**   • Compress at 100/minute   • Once advanced airway in place, give continuous compressions at 100/minute without pause for ventilation AND ventilate at 8-10 per minute.   • Minimize interruptions in compressions   • Rescuers should switch ventilation and compression roles every 2 minutes

↘

Check Rhythm: Is Shockable Rhythm (Ventricular Fibrillation OR Ventricular Tachycardia) Present?

↙   ↘

Shockable rhythm • Give one shock • Restart CPR immediately for five cycles		**Non shockable rhythm** • Restart CPR immediately for 5 cycles • Check rhythm q 5 cycles

During rhythm recheck (once advanced cardiac care available)

↙   ↘

Shockable rhythm See ventricular fibrillation & tachycardia page 4		**Nonshockable rhythm** See PEA, asystole page 5

[1] AED – Automatic External Defibrillator

Adult Advanced Resuscitation
Pulseless Cardiac Arrest/Ventricular Fibrillation & Tachycardia

Pulseless Cardiac Arrest

- See Basic Resuscitation - **Page 3**.
- Administer O$_2$, intubate, & attach monitor and defibrillator as soon as possible – without delaying compressions

Check Rhythm ↓

Is rhythm SHOCKABLE? Ventricular Fibrillation (VF) or Ventricular Tachycardia (VT) or **NONSHOCKABLE:** Asystole or Pulseless Electrical Activity (PEA). IF Asystole or PEA occurs at any time – **SEE Page 5** management

VT/VF present ↓

- Administer 1 Shock: (1) Manual biphasic @ 120-200 Joules (J) OR (2) AED which delivers device specific shock OR (3) Monophasic shock @ 360 J.
- Resume CPR for five cycles, then recheck Rhythm

VT/VF still present ↓

- Continue **CPR** while defibrillator is charging
- Administer 1 **Shock**: (1) manual biphasic (same as first shock [120-200J] or higher OR (2) AED - delivers device specific shock OR (3) Monophasic @ 360 J
- Resume **CPR** immediately after shock
- When Intravenous (IV) line or Intraosseous (IO) needle is available, give **vasopressor** during CPR either before or after the shock. Vasopressors include:
  - **Epinephrine** 1 mg IV or IO repeated q 3-5 minutes OR
  - **Vasopressin** 40 Units IV or IO to replace 1st or 2nd dose of epinephrine
- Recheck rhythm after 5 cycles of CPR

VT/VF still present ↓

- Continue **CPR** while defibrillator is charging
- Administer 1 **Shock**: (1) manual biphasic (same as first shock [120-200J] or higher OR (2) AED - delivers device specific shock OR (3) Monophasic @ 360 J
- Resume **CPR** immediately after shock
- Consider antiarrhythmics (below) during CPR either before or after the shock.
  - **Amiodarone** - 300 mg IV or IO X 1 dose. Consider additional 150 mg IV or IO
  - **Lidocaine** – 1 to 1.5 mg/kg IV or IO X 1 dose, then 0.5 to 0.75 mg/kg IV or IO every 5-10 minutes to a maximum of 3 doses or 3 mg/kg.
  - **Consider magnesium** – (if Torsades de pointes) – 1-2 g IV/IO over 5-20 min.

↓

- Once return of spontaneous circulation, treat underlying etiology (See page 5), consider amiodarone infusion 1mg/min X 6 hours plus 0.5 mg/min over 18 hours OR lidocaine 1-4 mg/min (depending upon which antiarrhythmic was used)

Adult Advanced Resuscitation
Asystole/Pulseless Electrical Activity[1]
(PEA = rhythm on monitor, without detectable pulse)

Pulseless Cardiac Arrest
• See Basic Resuscitation - **Page 3.** • Administer O_2, intubate, & attach monitor and defibrillator as soon as possible – without delaying compressions

Check Rhythm ↓

Is rhythm SHOCKABLE? Ventricular Fibrillation (VF) or Ventricular Tachycardia (VT) – IF SHOCKABLE RHYTHM, see **Page 4**. If **NONSHOCKABLE:** Asystole or Pulseless Electrical Activity (PEA) see below.

Asystole/PEA ↓

• Resume CPR immediately for 5 cycles
• When Intravenous (IV) line or Intraosseous (IO) needle is available, give **vasopressor** during CPR either before or after the shock. Vasopressors include:
   o <u>**Epinephrine**</u> - 1 mg IV or IO repeated q 3-5 minutes OR
   o <u>**Vasopressin**</u> - 40 Units IV or IO to replace 1st or 2nd dose of epinephrine.
   o <u>**Atropine**</u> – Consider 1 mg IV or IO for asystole or slow PEA rate, repeat every 3-5 minutes up to 3 doses.

Give 5 cycles of CPR ↓

• Recheck rhythm • **SHOCKABLE** rhythm (VF/pulseless VT), see page 4 • **NONSHOCKABLE** rhythm: If asystole return to box above, If electrical activity, check pulse. If no pulse go to box above.

During Resuscitation ↓

Review for most frequent causes and treat accordingly	
• Hypovolemia	• Tablets/toxins (drug OD, ingestion)
• Hypoxia	• Tamponade, cardiac
• Hydrogen ion – acidosis	• Tension pneumothorax
• Hyper/Hypo K+, other metabolic	• Thrombosis, coronary
• Hypoglycemia	• Thrombosis, pulmonary
• Hypothermia	• Trauma

[1] Pacing is not recommended for asystole. Norepinephrine and IV fluids are not recommended for cardiac arrest.

Pulseless PEDIATRIC Cardiac Arrest (AGE ≤ 8 YEARS)

- **Provide CPR**
- **Provide O_2, attach monitor, defibrillator**
- **Estimate weight using Broselow-Luten tape**
- **Assess rhythm**

VF/Pulseless VT[1]

Defibrillation
- Shock once at 2J/kg or
- Use AED > 1 year old

Resume CPR
for 5 cycles (2 minutes)

If VT/pulseless VT persist
- Shock once at 4J/kg or
- Use AED > 1 year old

- Resume CPR
- Give **epinephrine[3]** IV or IO at 0.01 mg/kg or via ETT at 0.1 mg/kg

After **5** cycles of CPR, recheck rhythm.

If VT/pulseless VT persist
- Shock once @ 4J/kg or
- Use AED > 1 year old

- Consider one of following
  1. **Amiodarone** 5 mg/kg IV/IO
  2. **Lidocaine** 1 mg/kg IV/IO
  3. **Magnesium** 25-50 mg/kg IV or IO (max 2 grams) if Torsades de pointes present

---

During CPR
- Give 15 compressions, then 2 breaths (if 2 person CPR)
- Secure airway and confirm placement (e.g. visualization followed by capnographic waveform analysis)
- After intubation, perform CPR without pausing for breaths (8-10 breaths/min) via ETT

Search for and treat causes of cardiac arrest
Hypovolemia, Hypoxia, Hydrogen ion (acidosis),Hypo/ Hyperkalemia, Hypoglycemia, Hypothermia, Toxins, Tamponade,Tension pneumo- thorax, Trauma, Thrombosis (coronary or pulmonary)

PEA[2] or asystole

- Resume CPR
- Give **epi[3]** IV or IO at 0.01 mg/kg (0.1 mg/kg of 10,000) or endotracheal at 0.1 mg/kg (0.1 ml/kg of 1:1,000)
- Repeat q3-5 min

Resume CPR
for 5 cycle (2 min)
- If pulseless VT or VF, see VT/VF algorithm to left

After meds, continue CPR for 5 cycles (2 min) and recheck rhythm.
If VT/Pulseless VF persists, resume CPR, rechecking rhythm every 2 min followed by shock and administering epi q 3-5 min & antiarrhythmics.
If asystole/PEA, treat per PEA/Asystole algorithm.

---

1. -VF – ventricular fibrillation, VT – ventricular tachycardia

2 PEA – pulseless electrical activity

3 Give epinephrine (epi) q 3-5 min. Consider higher dose (0.1mg/kg) administered IV or IO only in exceptional circumstances   (e.g. β blocker overdose)

Acid Base Disorders

Anion Gap	• $Na^+ - (Cl^- + HCO_3^-)$ *Normal* = 8-16 mEq/L
Osmolal gap	• measured – calculated osmolality *Normal* = 0-10 mOsm/L
Calculated Osmolality	• $2 \times Na^+ + (glucose/18) + (BUN/2.8) + (ethanol/4.6) + (methanol/2.6) + (ethylene\ glycol/5) + (acetone/5.5) + (isopropanol/5.9)$

Causes of ↑Anion Gap	Causes of ↓Anion Gap	Causes of ↑Osmol Gap
Methanol	Lactate	Lithium, bromide	Alcohols (methanol,
Uremia	Ethanol, ethylene	Multiple myeloma	ethylene glycol,
Diabetes	glycol	Albumin loss in	isopropanol)
Paraldehyde	Salicylates,	nephrotic syndrome	Sugar (glycerol, mannitol)
Iron, INH	starvation		Ketones (acetone)

	Primary Disorder	Normal Compensation
Acid Base Rules of Compensation	Metabolic Acidosis	$PCO_2 = (1.5 \times HCO_3^- + 8) \pm 2$
	Acute Respiratory Acidosis	↑ΔHCO_3^- = $(0.1 \times \Delta PCO_2$↑$)$
	Chronic Respiratory Acidosis	↑ΔHCO_3^- = $(0.4 \times \Delta PCO_2$↑$)$
	Metabolic Alkalosis	$PCO_2 = (0.9 \times HCO_3^- + 9) \pm 2$
	Acute Respiratory Alkalosis	↓ΔHCO_3^- = $(0.2 \times \Delta PCO_2$↓$)$
	Chronic Respiratory Alkalosis	↓ΔHCO_3^- = $(0.4 \times \Delta PCO_2$↓$)$

Anaphylaxis

MANAGEMENT OF ANAPHYLAXIS

Airway	Administer 100% O_2 & consider early intubation for airway edema
Cardiac	Apply cardiac monitor, & pulse oximeter, assess vitals frequently
Skin	Remove stinger, apply ice. Epinephrine (0.1-0.3 mg of 1:1,000) SC local to site if not an end organ (finger, toe, nose).
GI	Consider charcoal 50 g po for ingested allergen

Drugs	Dose	Route	Indications
epinephrine	0.01 mg/kg[1]	SC/IM	mild to moderate symptoms
		IV	airway compromise, severe hypotension IV dose – (see page 32 for mixture , use only for SEVERE life threat [1])
normal saline	20 ml/kg	IV	hypotension
Solu-Medrol	2 mg/kg	IV	moderate/severe symptoms
Benadryl	1 mg/kg	IV/IM	moderate/severe symptoms (max 50 mg)
cimetidine	5 mg/kg	IV/IM	if no wheezing (bronchoconstricts)
glucagon	2-5 mg	IV	if patient taking a β-blocker
albuterol	2.5 mg	nebulized	bronchospasm
racemic epi.	0.2-0.4 ml	nebulized	stridor (2.25% solution)

[1]Use with extreme caution as severe life-threatening complications can occur.

Anesthesia & Airway Management

Laryngeal Mask Airway (LMA) sizes					
Mask size	Weight	Age	LMA length	LMA cuff volume	Largest ETT
1	< 5 kg	< 0.5 yr	10 cm	4 ml	3.5 mm
1.5	5-10	< 1	10	5-7	4
2	6.5-20	0.5-5	11.5	7-10	4.5
2.5	20-30	5-10	12.5	14	5
3	30-60	10-15	19	15-20	6
4	60-80	> 15	19	25-30	6.5
5	> 80	> 15	19	30-40	7

Largest sized ET tube (int. diameter) that can pass through LMA for blind insertion

Rapid Sequence Intubation - Preparation

- ready 2 wall suction devices with Yankauer tips, check laryngoscope light
- select appropriate ET tube (7-7.5 mm internal diameter for adult females and 7.5-8 mm for males) and back-up 1 size smaller with stylet, check ET cuff
- raise bed to comfortable height (e.g., patient's nose at intubator's xiphoid)
- prepare alternate airway plan: (eg. LMA <u>above</u>, bougie, cricothyrotomy)
- ensure pulse oximeter and cardiac monitor attached and working
- specify personnel for (1) cricoid pressure, (2) neck immobilization if trauma, (3) handling ET tube, (4) watching O_2 sat & cardiac monitors, and (5) medications
- position head - sniffing position if no trauma, in-line stabilization if trauma
- draw up all drugs in syringes and ensure secure IV access is available
- preoxygenate with 100% oxygen for at least 3-4 minutes (if possible)
- perform Sellick maneuver (cricoid pressure)

Medication

- lidocaine 1.5 mg/kg IV if head injured to blunt ICP response to laryngoscopy
- defasciculating agent (optional) if succinylcholine given (then wait 1.5-2 min)
- administer sedating, then paralyzing agent IV (see page 9)

Drugs for Rapid Sequence Intubation

Agent	Dose IV	Onset	Key Properties
Defasciculating drug	(mg/kg)	(min)	Defasciculation (optional)
rocuronium[1]	0.06	2	tachycardia, mild histamine release
succinylcholine	0.1	< 1	↑ICP, GI, and eye pressures
vecuronium	0.01	2.5-5	minimal tachycardia
Sedating drug	(mg/kg)	(min)	
etomidate[2]	0.3-0.4	1	minimal blood pressure decrease
fentanyl	2-10 µg/kg	1	↑ICP, chest wall rigidity
ketamine	1-2	< 1	↑BP, ICP, GI, eye pressures
midazolam	0.1-0.3	2	causes hypotension
propofol	1-2.5	< 1	hypotension
thiopental	3-5	< 1	hypotension, bronchospasm
Paralyzing drug	(mg/kg)	(min)	
succinylcholine[3]	1-2	< 1	↑ICP, ↑ K+, ↑ GI and eye pressures
rocuronium	0.6-1.2	2	tachycardia, mild histamine release
vecuronium	0.15 - 0.25	2.5-5	prolonged action

[1]→[2]→[3] Standard drug sequence if no contraindications exist

Steps to Perform After Intubation	1. Check tube placement (CO_2 detector, esophageal detector device). Other methods including exam can be inaccurate. 2. Inflate cuff, then release cricoid pressure. 3. Normal depth of ET tube (cm) is ~3 X ET (at incisors) 4. Reassess patient's BP, pulse, and pulse oximetry. 5. Obtain CXR to verify correct ET depth (between T2-T4). 6. Sedate and consider long acting paralytics.

Guidelines for Initiating Mechanical Ventilation in Adults

Item	Initial Setting	Comments
Mode	Assist control	Ventilator assists if patient breathes on own
	Controlled,	Patient cannot breathe on own (e.g. paralyzed)
	IMV, SIMV	Set rate that allows patient to breathe on own
Tidal Volume	10-12 ml/kg	5-7 ml/kg if ↑peak airway pressures (e.g. asthma)
Rate	12-14/minute	
FiO_2	50-100%	Reduce as soon as possible to < 50%
PEEP	None	Start at 5 cm H_2O if paO_2 < 60 & FiO_2 ≥ 50%
I:E	1:2	Reverse ratio of ≥ 2:1 for ARDS, pulmonary edema
Insp. flow	50L/min	If too slow, causes inadequate exhalation
Insp. pause	None	Leads to even ventilation, and air trapping
Peak pressure	50 cm H_2O	Start at 20-30 if pressure cycled ventilator
Exp. retard	None	May prevent premature collapse of airway

Visit (1) www.bt.cdc.gov for updates re: biologic/chemical agents, (2) www.cdc.gov/other.htm#states or www.astho.org/state.html for state health departments, (3) www.orau.gov/reacts/care.htm or Call (615) 576-1004 re: radiation exposure. CDC Bioterrorism Preparedness and Response Center 1-770-488-7100

General rules – Gown, gloves, HEPA filter masks protect vs. most biological agents while soap/water removes most agents from skin. Hypochlorite (0.1%) bleach removes most contaminants from objects (do not use on skin unless VX exposure).

Anthrax – *Incubation* –Skin exposure leads to symptoms in a few days. Inhalation exposure leads to symptoms in < 1 week with possibility of symptoms occurring 2 months after exposure (and theoretically up to 100 days). *Features* – Initially patients develop fever/chills (> 95%), nausea/vomiting (80%), myalgia/headache (50% each), minimally-nonproductive cough (90%), then sweats, chest pain (60%), shortness of breath (80%), abdominal pain (30%), and shock. Rhinorrhea (~10%) & sore throat (20%) are rare. Skin - edema, then pruritic macule/papule, ulcer, painless, depressed eschar, lymphangitis, painful lymphadenopathy, *Diagnosis* – initial CXR-wide mediastinum (~70%), effusion (~80%), Wright or Gram stain blood or CSF with gram positive bacilli, positive blood cultures, or ELISA for toxin. *Chemoprophylaxis* (1) ciprofloxacin 500 mg PO BID X 60 d OR (2) doxycycline 100 mg PO BID X 60 (3) if organism penicillin sensitive, may switch to amoxicillin 500 mg PO TID X 60 d. If extremely high inhalation exposure, the CDC lists alternate options of above antibiotics for total of 100 days with or without vaccination (3 doses over 4 weeks). Ciprofloxacin or amoxicillin is recommended in exposed pregnant women. Switch to penicillin or amoxicillin once sensitivity known. *Treatment* for inhalational, GI, or oropharyngeal: (1) ciprofloxacin 400 mg IV q 12 hours. OR (2) doxycycline 100 mg IV q 12 h [do not use if meningitis possible] **PLUS** 1 or 2 of following agents: clindamycin, rifampin, vancomycin, penicillin, ampicillin, chloramphenicol, imipenem, or clarithromycin. Switch to combined [(1) or (2) above plus added agent(s)] oral antibiotics when clinically appropriate and continue antibiotics for total of 60 days (IV and PO combined). Steroids are a recommended option for patients with severe edema or meningitis.

Blistering Agents – Mustard gas - Severe skin, lung, or eye damage with delayed blisters up to 4-12 hours. Mustard passes through clothes without burning & through living tissue without symptoms for hours. Smell - mustard, onion, or garlic. Skin is red & blisters form late and skin initially may only look like 1st or 2nd degree burn. Airway irritation is prominent early. *Treat* First decontaminate and remove all clothing, jewelry. Remove skin droplets by blotting, cleanse with soap and water or chloramine solution. IV N-acetylcysteine may decontaminate systemically. Treat skin injury as chemical burn, with irrigation, topical antibiotics. Mild to moderate eye exposures may irrigate with 2.5% sodium thiosulfate. **Lewisite** - immediate burn eyes, nose, & skin (flushed). Treat by decontaminating & using dimercaprol.

Botulinum – <u>*Onset*</u> – 1-4 days. *Features* – afebrile, descending symmetric flaccid paralysis starts at cranial nerves. Normal mental status. 4D's: Dry mouth, dysarthria, dysphonia, and dysphagia are prominent. Respiratory failure ± in 24 hours. <u>*Diagnosis*</u> – Check gag, cough reflexes, inspiratory force, oxygen saturation. Consult local and state health department (page 10). Nasal swab ELISA or Serum, food bioassay. Gastric or stool samples may be tested if airborne or food borne. <u>*Treatment*</u> – Supportive, wash skin with soap/H_2O. Cleanse objects with 0.1% hypochlorite (bleach) solution. Trivalent (vs. A,B,C) or US Army heptavalent (vs. A to G) antitoxin (equine) may prevent progression. 1st, skin test with 0.2 ml diluted in 2 ml NS SC. If not allergic, dilute 10 ml vial with 90 ml NS and administer slow IV. If allergic, desensitize as per Crotalidae antivenin page 59-60.

Brucellosis –aerosol or food source <u>*Incubation*</u> – 1-4 weeks. <u>*Features*</u> – fever, headache, fatigue, colitis, hepatitis, arthritis, lymph nodes, osteomyelitis, epididy-moorchitis, endocarditis <u>*Diagnosis*</u> – blood & bone marrow culture, or serology. <u>*Prophylaxis*</u> –doxycycline 100 mg PO BID or ciprofloxacin 500 mg PO BID X 3 weeks. <u>*Treatment*</u> – (1) doxycycline 100 mg PO BID + rifampin 600-900 mg PO qd X 6 weeks OR (2) doxycycline X 6 weeks + streptomycin 1 g IM q 12h X 3 weeks.

Cyanide – colorless, inhale > ingest, bitter almond smell. H/A, dyspnea, HTN, ↑ HR then apnea, ↓BP, ↓ HR, seizure, dysrhythmias, cell death. Retinal veins cherry red. Labs – ↑ anion gap acidosis (lactate), venous pO_2 > 40 mm Hg. Treat (1) 100% O_2, (2) antidote kit (2a) inhale amyl nitrate 30 sec/min until IV meds ready; (2b) Na nitrate (10%) 0.33 ml/kg (10ml/300 mg max) IV. Use less if anemic. May ↓BP and induce methemoglobinemia (goal MetHb ≤ 25%); (2c) Na+ thiosulfate (25%) 1.65 ml/kg (12.5 g/50 ml max) IV, (3) Hyperbaric O_2 and hydroxycobalamin (B12) IV may also be useful.

Nerve Agents – [**GF**, **Sarin (GB)**, **Soman (GD)**, **Tabun (GA)**, **VX**, **Substance 33 (V-gas)**] –inhaled & dermally absorbed cholinesterase inhibitors (organophosphates). VX may persist on scene for weeks. Symptoms: CNS Δ (delirium, confusion, resp. depression, seizures), muscarinic (SLUDGE; salivate, lacrimate, urinate, defecation, GI, emesis, & miosis, bronchoconstrict, ↓HR) & nicotinic (muscles weak, HTN, ↑HR, ± mydriasis). Manage (1) decontaminate (rescuers wear protection) dermally with soap and water. Since hydrolysis converts VX into a longer lasting and toxic metabolic some experts recommend using 0.1% bleach (diluted hypochlorite household solution) to topically decontaminate VX. Avoid abrading skin.,(2) resp support (3) high dose atropine, (4) pralidoxime (esp. Sarin, VX, not Soman), See page 161 for dose. (5) Bispyridinium oximes or H oximes (e.g. obidoxime, HI-6) may reactivate aged cholinesterase that is resistant to pralidoxime. (esp. useful if Soman)

Phosgene – smells like newly mowed hay. Inhalation causes irritation to eyes, nose, skin with tissue damage in minutes. Chest tightness, difficulty breathing & delayed pulmonary edema occur (2-24 hours). A 24-48 hr period of latency after initial irritant or asymptomatic phase may occur. Decontaminate skin with water irrigation. Remove clothing. Medical personnel involved in topical decontamination require activated charcoal protective mask. Observe for 6 hours due to latency. Treat supportively.

Phosgene oxime (CX) is a urticariant/nettle gas that is topically absorbed and produces immense dermal pain penetrating to muscle layer. It penetrates garments and rubber acting rapidly. The skin is initially gray, blanched, then severe itching, hives, and blisters. Blanched area forms wheals that turn brown in 24 hours, forming eschar. CX also irritates eyes & lungs (ARDS). Decontaminate skin with water, or M291 military decontamination kit. Otherwise treat supportively.

PFIB (perfluoroisobutylene) gas can be made from heated *Teflon* and causes similar picture/more toxicity than phosgene. Initial eye, airway, chest irritation with early or delayed pulmonary edema after latent period. Shivering, sweating, fever, and tachypnea may occur similar to metal fume fever. Medical personnel require positive pressure air respiratory (charcoal respirator is inadequate). Ventilate with air to decontaminate and do not irrigate with water if PFIB exposure as this results in hydrofluoric acid formation. Observe for six hours due to latency. Treat supportively.

Plague – *Onset* 1-6 days. *Features* – bubonic (malaise, fever, purulent lymphadenitis), sepsis, or pneumonic (esp. weaponized) plague. Weaponized symptoms – fever, cough, dyspnea, hemoptysis, only rare cervical buboes. GI upset, vomiting, diarrhea common. CXR – patchy/consolidated pneumonia. *Diagnosis* – Wright-Giemsa or gram stain of sputum, node, or blood (gram negative, bipolar/safety pin shaped) or culture of blood, lymph node aspirate or sputum. Specific tests (e.g. PCR) available at state health departments (page 10) *Chemoprophylaxis* (1) doxycycline 100 mg PO BID OR (2) ciprofloxacin 500 mg PO BID X 7 days. *Treatment* – (1) streptomycin 1 g IM q 12 hours OR (2) gentamicin 5 mg/kg IV/IM q day OR (3) gentamicin 2 mg IV load, then 1.7 mg/kg IV q 8 hours OR (4) doxycycline 100 mg IV q 12 hours OR (5) ciprofloxacin 400 mg IV q 12 hours – continue for 10 days total. Gentamicin dosed as above preferred in pregnant women although doxycycline or ciprofloxacin may be used as alternatives. May switch to oral agents upon clinical improvement.

Q fever – *Coxiella burnetii* Incubation 10-40 days, *Features* – influenza-like with fever, atypical pneumonia/hilar nodes, hepatitis. *Diagnosis* – ELISA, *Treatment* – ciprofloxacin or doxycycline X 15-21 days [anthrax dose], macrolides also may be effective.

Radiation – *Features* - acute radiation syndrome – 1st: nausea, vomiting, diarrhea, fatigue X 1-2 days, ± burns (±7-10 days to blister) 2nd symptom free latency (absent if > 1000 rads) 3rd overt symptoms: GI (vomiting, diarrhea, bleed, sepsis), CNS (confusion, edema), Heme (↓WBC [lymphocytes] Hb & platelets ± delayed 2-3 weeks if low dose) *Treatment* – Protective clothes, radiation monitor for medical personnel. Treat trauma, externally decontaminate. Admit if ≥ 200 rads. If no symptoms 1st 24 hours, exposure is < 75 rads. CBC& diff. q 6-8 hours. Reverse isolation, anti-emetics, colony stimulation factor, stem cell, platelet & Hb transfusion, tissue & blood typing (family/marrow transplant). Prophylactic antibiotics, antivirals, anti-fungals prn.

Radioactive fallout from radioactive iodine (e.g. nuclear reactor) causes exposure via inhalation, or ingestion (e.g. cow's milk) resulting in cancer (esp. thyroid). Depending on thyroid exposure in rads, potassium iodide (KI) is recommended by CDC.

Population	Predicted thyroid exposure	Daily KI[1] dose
Adults over 40 years	> 500 rad	130 mg
Adults > 18 to 40 years	≥ 10	130 mg
Pregnancy or lactating	≥ 5	130 mg
> 12 to 18 years (if ≥ 70 kg, treat as adult)	≥ 5	65 mg
> 3 to 12 years	≥ 5	65 mg
> 1 mo to 3 years (dilute in milk, formula, H₂0)	≥ 5	32 mg
0-1 months	≥ 5	16 mg

[1]Do not give if known iodine sensitive, dermatitis herpetiformis, or hypocomplementemic vasculitis & use cautiously if thyroid disease. KI protects only thyroid gland from radioiodines, offers no protection from external radiation, does not protect from effect of exposure to other radioactive materials. KI lasts 24 h, use daily until no risk

www.fda.gov/cder/guidance/index.htm

Ricin (or **Abrin**)– type II ribosome inactivation from castor beans/seeds. <u>Onset</u> – 4-8 h after inhaled. <u>Features</u> - ingestion - GI distress, necrosis, hepatitis; <u>inhalation</u> – pulm necrosis, shock. Metabolic acidosis, hepatitis, hematuria, renal failure. <u>Diagnosis</u> – Serum or resp. secretion ELISA, <u>Treat</u>– remove clothes, cleans objects with 0.1% hypochlorite (bleach), wash skin with soap/water, provide supportive care, oral charcoal if PO ingested. If injected, excision of area may be useful.

Smallpox – orthopox virus. <u>Incubation</u> – 7-17 days. <u>Features</u> – fever, headache, backache. Maculapapular rash face > mouth/pharynx, mucosa & arms/legs, palms, soles (*Varicella* causes rash on trunk > other areas, at different stages, & no palm/sole involvement). 1-2 days rash is vesicular, then pustular. Round/tense pustules deeply embedded with crusting on 8-9th day. All lesions evolve at same rate. A rapidly progressive form with sepsis, skin petechiae, hemorrhage can occur as well as a malignant form with abrupt onset, with flattened confluent skin lesions never progressing to pustules. <u>Diagnosis</u> - Vesicle/pustule fluid or scabs can be examined by electron microscopy. <u>Prevention</u> - Vaccine may prevent disease if given within 3-4 days of exposure. Vaccine reactions including generalized or progressive vaccinia, eczema vaccinatum and periocular infections are treated with vaccinia immune globulin 0.6 ml/kg divided over 24-36 hours since volume is 42 ml in a 70 kg adult. May repeat in 2-3 days. <u>Treatment</u> - decontaminate surfaces with 0.1% hypochlorite (bleach) or quaternary ammonia. Isolate if ill and provide support.

Staphylococcal enterotoxin B – inhaled or ingested. <u>Onset</u> – 1-12 hours <u>Features</u> – sudden fever (often ≥ 40°C/104°F) for up to 5 days, headache, chills, dyspnea, vomiting, diarrhea (if swallow aerosol), & cough up to 4 weeks. CXR - normal, ARDS can develop. <u>Diagnosis</u> – Abrupt onset of fever, respiratory symptoms in large numbers of exposed presenting at same time, normal CXR, & nonprogression. Toxin - difficult to ID. Nasal swab ELISA in 1st 24 h may be +. <u>Treat:</u> supportively

Trichothecene Mycotoxins – fungal toxins (e.g. yellow rain) inhibit protein & DNA synthesis, and destroy cells. _Onset_ – minutes to hours. _Features_ -Skin damage (blisters). Ingestion: vomiting, bloody diarrhea, and GI bleed. Inhalation: acute eye pain/red, tears, bloody rhinorrhea, hemoptysis + skin findings, ARDS, ↓ BP, bone marrow depression and sepsis. _Diagnosis_ – gas liquid chromatography blood, urine, stool, lung washings. _Treatment_ – supportive, ascorbic acid, dexamethasone, GI decontamination/lavage, eye (saline irrigation).

Tularemia – _Francisella tularensis_ (gram negative bacillus). _Incubation_ – 1-14 days. _Features_ –glandular (nodes without ulcer), ulceroglandular (indurated, punched out ulcers with lymphadenitis, draining nodes with 10-30% pneumonic). Pneumonic & septic tularemia are weaponized forms – influenza-like symptoms without pneumonia or atypical pneumonia, hilar nodes (not generalized mediastinal widening as in anthrax), effusion. Abdominal pain, vomiting, diarrhea predominate early. _Diagnosis_ – gram stain sputum (small gram negative coccobacilli), serology (ELISA), culture sputum, fasting gastric aspirate, pharyngeal washings. _Chemoprophylaxis_ – doxycycline 100 mg PO BID X 14 days OR ciprofloxacin 500 mg PO BID X 14 days. _Treat_ – (1) gentamicin 5 mg/kg IV/IM q 24 h X 10 days OR (2) streptomycin 1 g IM q 12 hours X 10 days OR (3) doxycycline 100 mg IV q 12 hours X 14 days OR (4) ciprofloxacin 400 mg IV q 12 hours X 10 days. Switch to oral medications when clinically improved.

Viral Encephalitides – (Venezuelan equine encephalitis/VEE, eastern/EEE & western equine/WEE) highly infectious by aerosol. _Incubation_ – VEE 2-6 days, EEE/WEE 7-14 days. _Features_ – fever, headache, myalgias. VEE causes symptoms in most. Only 0.5-4 % have neurologic involvement. EEE will kill 50-75%. _Diagnosis_ – ↓ serum WBC count, CSF – pleocytosis/lymphocytosis, acutely serum IgM antibodies, ELISA, & hemagglutination-inhibiting antibodies are positive by 2nd week. _Treatment_ – no person-person transmission, provide supportive care.

Viral Hemorrhagic fevers (VHF) –due to a variety of RNA viruses (e.g. Marburg, Ebola, yellow fever). _Incubation_ – 4-21 days. _Features_ – fever, myalgias, prostration, early conjunctival injection, mild hypotension, flushing, petechial hemorrhages. Variety of skin rashes occur –online pictures are available at www.jama.ama-assn.org/ JAMA 2002; 287: 2391. Later jaundice, DIC picture with hepatitis, renal failure and CV collapse. _Diagnosis_ – ↓ WBCs count (↑WBCs with Lassa fever), anemia or hemoconcentration, ↓ platelets, ↑LFTs, ↑PT/PTT, ↓ fibrinogen. Diagnose by ELISA, or PCR state or federal lab. _Prophylaxis_ – yellow fever vaccine is available but disease onset would occur before vaccine becomes effective. Health care workers require personal air purifying respirators or N-95 mask, negative isolation rooms, complete torso, leg, shoe, face coverings, and goggles. All medical equipment should be dedicated to single patient. Disinfect objects with 0.1% hypochlorites (bleach) _Treatment_ –If VHF due to unknown cause, arenavirus, or bunyavirus administer ribavirin 30 mg/kg IV (max 2 g), then 16 mg/kg (max 1 g) IV q 6 hours X 4 days, then 8 mg/kg IV (max 500 mg) q8 hours X 6 days. If mass casualties, load with ribavirin 2000 mg PO, followed by 600 mg PO BID (if > 75 kg) OR [400 mg PO q AM + 600 mg PO q PM (if ≤ 75 kg)] X 10 days. Otherwise, supportive care.

Burns and Burn Therapy

Estimation of Total Body Surface Area Burned

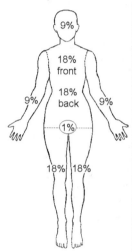

Admission and Transfer Criteria for Patients with Significant Burns

Admission Criteria[1]

Burn TBSA ≥ 15% (2nd + 3rd degree)
Burn TBSA ≥ 10% (age > 50 years)
Burn TBSA ≥ 2-5% (3rd degree)
Burns to hands, feet, face, perineum
Minor chemical burn
Associated carbon monoxide poisoning
Inadequate family support or known or suspected abuse
Severe underlying medical disease (e.g. emphysema, coronary artery disease, diabetes, renal insufficiency)

Transfer to Burn Center[1]

Burn TBSA ≥ 25% (2nd + 3rd degree)
Burn TBSA ≥ 20% (age > 50 years)
Burn TBSA ≥ 10% (3rd degree)
3rd degree hands, feet, face, perineum
Major chemical or electrical burn
Respiratory tract injury
Associated major trauma
Circumferential limb burns

[1]TBSA - total body surface area

Fluid Resuscitation in Burn Victims

Parkland formula	• Lactated ringers 4 ml/kg/%burn TBSA[1] in 1st 24 hours + maintenance fluid, with ½ over 1st 8 h, & ½ over next 16 h
Alternatives	• *Amended Parkland formula*: for ED stays < 8 hours. IV rate over maintenance (ml/h) = [weight(kg) X burn TBSA%] ÷ 4 • *Carvajal's formula*: Carvajal's solution 5,000 ml/m² of burn + maintenance 2000 ml/m² in 1st 24h, with ½ over the 1st 8 hours and ½ over the subsequent 16 hours.

[1]BSA = body surface area

BSA (m²) = ([Height (cm) X Weight (kg)] ÷ 3600)½ **OR**

BSA (m) = ([Height (inches) X Weight (pounds)] ÷ 3131)½

ECG Diagnosis of Arrhythmia, Blocks, and Medical Disorders

Normal Adult ECG (small box: 1 mm = 0.04 sec; large box: 5 mm = 0.20 sec)
- *P wave* - < 0.10 sec, ↑ in I, II, and ↓ in aVR.; *PR interval* - 0.12 - 0.20 sec.
- *QRS complex* - 0.05-0.10 seconds; normally ↑ in I, II, V5, V6; ↓ in aVR,V1; transition zone in V3; ↑ or ↓ in aVL, aVF,III; left chest leads height is < 27 mm.
- *Q wave*- normally < 0.04 seconds, and < 25% height of following R.
- *QT interval* - 0.34-0.42 seconds or 40% of RR interval
- *QTc* (corrected QT) = QT interval/square root of R-R.   Normal < 0.47 seconds.
- *T wave* - ↑ in I, V6, and ↓ in aVR; Normal ↓ T waves may be found in III, aVF, aVL,V1 : Abnormal ↓ T waves may signify LVH (esp V6), LBBB, ischemia, MI.
- *Axis* : Normal: -30 degrees to +100 degrees. *Left axis deviation* (LAD): -30 to -90 degrees. *Right axis deviation* (RAD): +100 to +180 or -90 to -180 degrees.

Conduction Blocks
- *1st degree AV block* - PR interval > 0.2 seconds, P precedes each QRS.
- *2nd degree AV block* - (type 1/Wenckebach) - increasing PR interval until QRS dropped. (type 2) - QRS dropped without increasing PR interval.
- *3rd degree AV block* - P and QRS are independent. Fixed P-P intervals.
- *Right bundle branch block (RBBB)* (1) QRS ≥ 0.12 sec (± 0.1-0.12 sec) (2) R-R'/R-S-R' in V1/V2 (3) ST-T opposite to terminal QRS (4) S in I, aVL,V5,V6.
- *Left bundle branch block (LBBB)* - (1) QRS ≥ 0.12 sec (2) R or R-R' in I, aVL, or V6; (3) negative wave (rS or QS) in V1, (4) no septal Q wave of 0.01 or 0.02 in I and V6. (5) ST-T waves directed opposite to the terminal 0.04 sec QRS.
- *Anterior Hemiblock* - LAD > - 45, QRS 0.10-0.12 sec, small Q in I, aVL; R in II, III, and aVF; terminal R in aVR.
- *Posterior Hemiblock* - RAD; QRS 0.10-0.12 sec; S in I; Q in II, III, aVF.

Hypertrophy
- *Right Atrial* - P > 2.5 mm in II or large diphasic P in V1 (tall initial phase)
- *Left Atrial* - diphasic P in V1 with large terminal downward phase.
- *Right Ventricular (RVH)* - RAD > 100, incomplete RBBB in V1; R>S - V1; R > 5 mm - V1; decreasing R in V1 to V4; ST depression + flipped T's V1-V3, ± RAH.
- *Left Ventricular (LVH)* – Romhilt and Estes criteria, Cornell criteria (page 17)

Romhilt & Estes Criteria for Left Ventricular Hypertrophy[1]	Points
QRS with largest R or S in limb leads ≥ 20 mm **or** S in V1 or V2 ≥ 30 mm **or** R in V5 or V6 ≥ 30 mm	3
ST-T downsloping without digitalis (3 points) or with digitalis (1 point)	1 or 3
Left atrial enlargement	3
Left axis deviation < 30 degrees or more	2
QRS duration > 0.9 seconds	1
Intrinsicoid deflection (onset QRS to apex R) in V5/V6 ≥ 0.05 sec.	1
Total points ≥ 5 = definite LVH, total points = 4 signifies probable LVH	

[1] 40-50% sensitivity, 80-90% specificity

Cornell Criteria for Diagnosing Left Ventricular Hypertrophy[1,2]
R in AVL + S in V3 ≥ 2.8 mV (males) & ≥ 2.0 mV (females)

[1] 42% sensitivity, 96% specificity

[2] R in AVL > 1.1 mV is also 97% specific for LVH

ECG Findings in Pericarditis

- ST segment elevation is typically diffuse involving ↑ in I, II, and III or at least 2 bipolar limb leads and precordial leads V1 through V6 or V2 through V6.
- ST depression is common in aVR, and may occur in II and V1. ST segment ↑ is typically concave upward and ≤ 5 mm in height. Pathologic Q waves are rare unless associated with MI. PR segment depression is common.
- Sequence of ST-T changes: (1) initial ST ↑, (2) ST returns to baseline before T waves flip (↓) (3) T wave ↓ is usually ≤ 5 mm (4) T waves normalize.
- Low voltage QRS or electrical alternans suggests pericardial fluid.
- ± Height of ST segment/T wave > 0.25 in V5, V6, or I.

ECG Findings in Medical Disorders

Disorder	Class ECG Findings (not necessarily most common)
CNS bleed	Diffuse deep T inversion, prominent U's, QT > 60% normal
COPD	RAD (negative lead I), overall low voltage, RAH ± RBBB
Pulmonary emboli	ST/T wave changes, RAD, RBBB. large S in I, Q in III, T in III
Hyperkalemia	Peaked T's, wide then flat P's, wide QRS and QT, sine wave
Hypokalemia	Flat T waves, U waves, U > T waves, ST depression
Calcium	High calcium - short QT, low calcium - long QT interval
Pericarditis	Flat/concave ST ↑, PR ↓, ↓ voltage
Digoxin effect	Downward curve of ST segment, flat/inverted T's, shorter QT
Digoxin toxicity	PVC's (60%), AV block (20%), Ectopic SVT (25%), V tach.
Hypothyroidism	Sinus bradycardia, low voltage, ST ↓, flat or inverted T waves
Hyperthyroidism	Sinus tachycardia

Myocardial injury and ischemia.

Location	ECG ST elevation or Q waves	Coronary Arteries involved
Anterior	V2-V4	Left anterior descending (LAD)
Anteroseptal	V1-V4	LAD
Anterolateral	V1-V6, I, aVL	LAD, diagonal
Inferior	II, III, aVF	Right coronary, circumflex
Lateral	I, aVL, V5, V6	Circumflex, diagonal
Posterior	large R -V1,V2,V3, reciprocal ST ↓	Right coronary artery
Posteriolat.	V6-V9	Right coronary artery

ST ↑ ≥ 1 mm = injury/infarction in 2 contiguous leads, Q > 0.04 sec = infarction

Typical ECG Findings in Acute MI

- Early on, a marked increase in R wave voltage may occur.
- Prominent (hyperacute) T waves with normal direction occur early (esp. > 5 mm). T waves are peaked and symmetric ~ church steeple (± wider than ↑K).
- ST segment elevation that is flat or convex > concave upward.
- Q waves > 0.04 sec other than leads aVR + V1 and T wave flattening/inversion.

Predictive Value of Initial ECG in Acute MI	Sensitivity	Specificity
• New Q waves or ST segment elevation	40%	> 90%
• Above or ST segment depression	75%	80%
• Any of above or prior ischemia/infarction changes	85%	76%
• Any of above or nonspecific ST-T changes	90%	65%

Ann Emerg Med 1990; 19: 1359

Diagnosis of Acute MI in Presence of Left Bundle Branch Block

Criteria for Diagnosis of Acute MI (Sgarbossa criteria)	Points
• ST segment elevation ≥ 1 mm concordant (same direction) as QRS	5
• ST segment depression ≥ 1 mm in leads V1, V2, or V3	3
• ST segment elevation ≥ 5 mm and discordant (opposite) with QRS	2

Total ≥ 3 is 36-78% sensitive, 90-96% specific for acute MI. *New Engl J Med* 1996;334: 481.

Most Common Causes of ST Segment Elevation in ED Chest Pain Patients

Disorder	Percent
• Left Ventricular Hypertrophy	25%
• Left Bundle Branch Block	15%
• Acute Myocardial Infarction	15%
• Benign Early Repolarization	12%
• Right Bundle Branch Block & Intraventricular conduction delay	5% each
• Ventricular Aneurysm	3%
• Pericarditis & Paced rhythm	1% each
• Undefined	17%

Am J Emerg Med 2001; 19:

Arrhythmias – Identification – See algorithm page 21, 24-26

- <u>Multifocal atrial tachycardia</u> - 3 or more different P waves, normal QRS complex and associated with COPD, hypoxia, digoxin or theophylline toxicity, or ASCVD.
- <u>Paroxysmal atrial tachycardia</u> - P's occur before each QRS with rate 150-250.
- <u>Paroxysmal supraventricular tachycardia</u> - Rate 120-250, narrow or wide QRS (if Bundle Branch Block or pre-excitation), P waves are visible or hidden in QRS
- <u>Atrial flutter</u> - atrial rate 200-400 saw tooth pattern (esp. leads II and III), common ventricular rate of 150 due to 2:1 block (with atrial rate of 300).
- <u>Atrial fibrillation</u> - highly irregular rhythm, no discernible P waves, ventricular rate may be rapid or slow depending on conduction.
- <u>Ventricular tachycardia</u> - ≥ 3 premature vent. beats in a row, broad QRS rhythm at 100-250/min. Fusion beats, AV dissociation, LAD, precordial concordance.
- <u>Ventricular fibrillation</u> (VF) - irregular chaotic baseline, no beats, no BP.
- <u>Torsades de pointes</u> - twisting QRS, prolonged QT interval, may progress to VF.

Differentiation of Wide Complex SVT from Ventricular Tachycardia

Feature	Suggests SVT	Suggests VT[1]
Age	< 35 years	> 50 years
Prior MI		95% specific for VT
Past Hx	Prior SVT	Angina, Congestive heart failure
Symptoms and BP	Not useful differentiator	Not useful differentiator
AV dissociation	Not applicable (n/a)	specific for VT
QRS duration	n/a	≥ 0.14 seconds (≥ 0.16 if LBBB)
QRS axis	n/a	-90 to ± 180 degrees (NW axis) or concordance in all precordial leads
V1 or V2 if LBBB	n/a	R > .03 sec, or > .07 sec to S nadir
V6 if LBBB	n/a	QR or QS
V1 if RBBB	triphasic QRS or R'>R	Monophasic R, QR, RS
V6 if RBBB	triphasic QRS	R/S < 1, QS, QR

[1] Absence of features suggesting VT DOES NOT imply SVT is more likely. No single feature is 100% accurate at differentiating between VT/SVT.

Emerg Med Clin N Am 1995; 13: 903.

Algorithm for Diagnosis of Wide Complex QRS Tachycardia

Is RS complex absent in all precordial leads?	Yes→	Ventricular tachycardia

No ↓

Is R to S interval > 100 ms (beginning of R to lowest point of S wave) in 1 precordial lead?	Yes→	Ventricular tachycardia

No ↓

Is Atrio-ventricular dissociation present?	Yes→	Ventricular tachycardia

No ↓

Morphology criteria for VT present both in precordial leads V1-V2 & V6 (see above table)	Yes→	Ventricular tachycardia

No ↓

SVT with aberrant conduction is likely

Sensitivity 99%, specificity 97%, in 1st study; Sensitivity 79-83%, specificity 43-70% in 2nd study. Accuracy lowered if on anti-dysrhythmics.

Circulation 1991; 83: 1649; Acad Emerg Med 2000; 7: 769.

Symptomatic **BRADYCARDIA** Management

Symptomatic Bradycardia

- Heart rate < 60 beats per minute AND
- Heart rate inadequate for clinical condition

↓

- Keep airway patent and assist breathing if needed
- Administer oxygen
- Monitor ECG, analyze rhythm, monitor blood pressure, and pulse oximetry
- Obtain IV access

↓

- Are the **signs or symptoms of decreased perfusion/shock** due to bradycardia? *Signs/symptoms of diminished perfusion include an acute altered mental status, persistent chest pain, ↓ BP or other signs/symptoms of shock*

Adequate perfusion ↓   ↓ Poor perfusion/shock

| Monitor patient |

↓

- Prepare for **transcutaneous pacing** – use immediately for high degree AV block (e.g. type 2 - 2nd degree, and 3rd degree AV block)
- **Epinephrine** – consider 2-10 mcg/min infusion OR **Dopamine** – consider 2-10 mcg/kg/min infusion while waiting for pacemaker or if pacing does not work.
- **Atropine** – consider administration of 0.5 mg IV while waiting for pacer. Repeat to a total dose of 3 mg. If does not work, begin pacing.
- **Prepare for transvenous pacing**
- **Treat underlying cause (see below)**
- **Cardiology consultation**

↙

IF PEA develops, See PEA management page 5.
Review for most frequent causes and treat accordingly.

- Hypovolemia
- Hypoxia
- Hydrogen ion – acidosis
- Hyper/Hypo K+, other metabolic
- Hypoglycemia
- Hypothermia

- Tablets/toxins (drug OD, ingestion)
- Tamponade, cardiac
- Tension pneumothorax
- Thrombosis, coronary
- Thrombosis, pulmonary
- Trauma

Tachycardia with pulse

- Keep airway patent, assist breathing, and support circulation if needed.
- Administer oxygen, secure airway (intubate if needed) and obtain IV access.
- Monitor ECG, analyze rhythm, monitor blood pressure, and pulse oximetry.
- Identify and treat Identifiable causes. (See last box page 20)

↓

- **Is Patient Unstable?** (new altered mentation, persistent chest pain, ↓BP, or other signs of shock). Rate related symptoms are uncommon if HR < 150/min.

Stable ↙	Unstable ↘
• Ensure IV access is present	• Immediately cardiovert-synchronized
• Obtain 12 leak EKG or rhythm strip	• Sedate beforehand if time permits
• Is the QRS width narrow (QRS < 12 seconds)?	• If PEA develops, see page 5.
	• Consider cardiology consult.

Narrow ↓   (If Wide Complex Tachycardia– See WCT box below) → ↘

- **Narrow Complex + Regular Rhythm** present - (1) Vagal maneuvers (2) Give adenosine 6 mg IV push, if do not convert, give 12 mg IV q 2 min X 2
  - ○ **If regular rhythm converts** – Reentry SVT was probably present. Observe for recurrence and treat recurrence with adenosine or longer acting AV node blocking drugs (e.g. diltiazem, β blockers)
  - ○ **If regular rhythm does not convert** – Possible atrial fluter, atrial or junctional tachycardia. Control rate (diltiazem or β blockers [caution if CHF or pulmonary disease). Treat underlying cause & consider cardiology consult.
- **Narrow Complex + Irregular Rhythm** – Probable atrial fibrillation or flutter or multifocal atrial tachycardia. Consider expert consultation and control rate using diltiazem or B blockers (caution if CHF or pulmonary disease)

↓ ↓ ↓ ↓ ↓ ↓ ↓ ↓

↙

Wide Complex Tachycardia (QRS ≥ 0. 12 seconds)

- **Regular Rhythm** – if ventricular tachycardia or uncertain rhythm
  - ○ **Amiodarone** – 150 mg IV over 10 min, repeat prn to max 2.2 g in 24 hours.
  - ○ **Elective synchronized cardioversion**
- **Regular Rhythm** – If SVT with aberrancy, give adenosine (see dosing above)
- **Irregular Rhythm** – If SVT with aberrancy, see narrow complex, irregular rhythm
- **Irregular Rhythm** – If pre-excitation atrial fibrillation (WPW). expert consultation advised. Avoid AV nodal blocking agents (adenosine, digoxin, diltiazem, verapamil). Consider **amiodarone** 150 mg IV over 10 minutes.
- **If recurrent polymorphic Ventricular Tachycardia** – consider expert consult.
- **If Torsades de pointes** – magnesium 1-2 g IV over 5-60 min + infusion.

Management of Atrial Fibrillation & Atrial Flutter

	Rate control[1]		Rhythm conversion[1]	
	Heart function preserved	*Impaired heart EF < 40%/CHF*	*< 48 hours duration*	*>48 hours or unknown*
Atrial Fibrillation or Atrial Flutter (AF)	If AF > 48 h use rate control drugs with extreme caution if not adequately anticoagulated Use only 1 of following[3]: Ca channel blocker (I) β blocker (I)	If AF > 48 h use rate control drugs with extreme caution if not adequately anticoagulated Use only 1 of following[3]: Digoxin (IIb) Diltiazem (IIb) Amiodarone(IIb)	**Consider** DC Cardioversion Use only 1 of following[3]: Amiodarone Ibutilide Flecainide Procainamide Propafenone (All of above are class IIa for this situation)	No DC CVS[2] Delayed CVS[1] anticoagulate X 3 weeks, CVS, anticoagulateX 4 more weeks Early CVS[1] 1st IV heparin + Echo to rule out atrial clot, then CVS within 24 h, + antico-agulate x 4week
Afib or flutter with Wolff Parkinson White	See AF > 48 h cautions above DC CVS **Or** 1 of following[3]: Amiodarone Flecainide Procainamide Propafenone Sotalol (All class IIb) Class III drugs Adenosine β blockers Ca blockers Digoxin	See AF > 48 h cautions above DC CVS **Or** Amiodarone (IIb)	DC CVS **Or** 1 of following[3]: Amiodarone Flecainide Procainamide Propafenone Sotalol (All of above are class IIb for this situation) Class III drugs Adenosine β blockers Ca blockers Digoxin	Anticoagulation as described above followed by DC CVS

[1] Class recommendations: Class I - definitely useful – Class IIa - accepted, safe, useful (intervention of choice), Class IIb - accepted, safe, useful (optional intervention), Class III – usually contraindicated, no benefit, may be harmful

[2] CVS – cardioversion

[3] See pages 30-34 for drug dosing

American College of Cardiology (ACC)/American Heart Association (AHA)
Guidelines for Managing Atrial Fibrillation/Flutter[1]

- <u>History and examination</u> to determine (1) type of AF (1st episode, paroxysmal, persistent or permanent), (2) onset 1st attack or 1st diagnosis, (3) frequency, duration, precipitants, prior methods of terminating, (4) prior response to drugs & (5) presence of other disease (cardiac ischemia, alcoholism, hyperthyroidism)

- <u>EKG</u> to assess arrhythmia, blocks, chamber, preexcitation, prior MI, and to measure and follow RR, QRS, and QT intervals, <u>CXR</u>, <u>Echocardiography</u> to evaluate valves, chambers, pericardium, RV pressures, clots, <u>Thyroid function</u> tests for 1st episode when rate difficult to control or if AF reoccurs unexpectedly. <u>Other tests</u> are indicated with specific scenarios: Holter monitor (adequacy of rate control), exercise test (suspected cardiac ischemia or type IC antiarrhythmic planned), transesophageal echo (stroke or systemic embolism), electrophysiologic study (clarify mechanism of wide QRS tachycardia, to identify atrial flutter or paroxysmal SVT, seek sites for ablation of AV conduction block/modification)

- <u>Heart Rate control</u> – (Recommended IV agents)
  - ◆ If congestive heart failure (CHF) is NOT present (and no contraindications) Class I agents for rate control: diltiazem, esmolol, metoprolol, propranolol, and verapamil. Digoxin is recommended Class IIa agent if no CHF.
  - ◆ If congestive heart failure is present, esmolol and digoxin are Class I agents for heart rate control. In this instance, diltiazem, metoprolol, propranolol, and verapamil are designated as Class IIb. (see pages 30-34 for dosing)
  - ◆ If accessory pathway (e.g. Wolf Parkinson White syndrome) suspected (e.g. wide QRS complex), IV procainamide or ibutilide are Class I recommendations for AF conversion to sinus rhythm. Amiodarone is a class II management alternative. In AF, avoid ß blockers, calcium channel blockers, digoxin if preexcitation (accessory pathway) is suspected.
  - ◆ Perform immediate electrocardioversion if acute paroxysmal AF and a rapid ventricular response associated with acute MI, symptomatic hypotension, angina or cardiac failure that does not respond promptly to drug therapy.
  - ◆ In patients requiring immediate cardioversion (chemical or electrical), administer heparin (or low molecular weight heparin) concurrently if time allows.

- <u>Anticoagulate</u> 1st with heparin (or low molecular weight heparin) all patients with AF > 48 hours, followed by oral anticoagulation for ≥3-4 weeks or longer.

- <u>Rhythm conversion</u> – Other than patients requiring immediate cardioversion, the timing, necessity, and techniques of conversion are complex (and controversial) and are left to consulting/admitting physicians.

[1] Class recommendations: Class I - definitely useful – Class IIa - accepted, safe, useful (intervention of choice), Class IIb - accepted, safe, useful (optional intervention)

AHA/ACC. *Circulation* 2001; 38: 1266.

Differential Diagnosis for narrow QRS tachycardia (< 120 milliseconds)

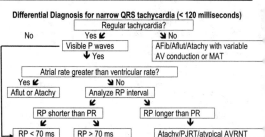

Afib – atrial fibrillation, Aflut – atrial flutter, Atachy – atrial tachycardia, AVRT - AV reciprocating tachycardia, AVNRT–AV nodal reciprocating tachycardia, MAT–multifocal atrial
tachycardia, PFRT – permanent junction reciprocating tachycardia, ms - milliseconds

Tachycardia Recognition & Response to Adenosine

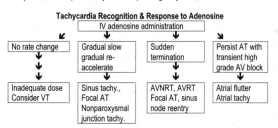

AT – atrial tachycardia, AV- atrioventricular node, VT – ventricular tachycardia, AVNRT –
AV nodal reciprocating tachycardia, AVRT – AV reciprocating tachycardia, tachy –
tachycardia   AHA/ACC *Circulation* 2003: 1871

Narrow Complex Supraventricular Tachycardia - Stable

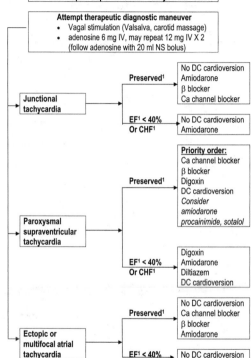

Attempt therapeutic diagnostic maneuver
- Vagal stimulation (Valsalva, carotid massage)
- adenosine 6 mg IV, may repeat 12 mg IV X 2
  (follow adenosine with 20 ml NS bolus)

Junctional tachycardia

Preserved[1]
No DC cardioversion
Amiodarone
β blocker
Ca channel blocker

EF[1] < 40% Or CHF[1]
No DC cardioversion
Amiodarone

Paroxysmal supraventricular tachycardia

Preserved[1]
Priority order:
Ca channel blocker
β blocker
Digoxin
DC cardioversion
Consider amiodarone procainimide, sotalol

EF[1] < 40% Or CHF[1]
Digoxin
Amiodarone
Diltiazem
DC cardioversion

Ectopic or multifocal atrial tachycardia

Preserved[1]
No DC cardioversion
Ca channel blocker
β blocker
Amiodarone

EF[1] < 40% Or CHF[1]
No DC cardioversion
Amiodarone
Diltiazem

Preserved – preserved cardiac function, EF – Ejection fraction, CHF – congestive heart failure. See pages 30-34 for drug dosing

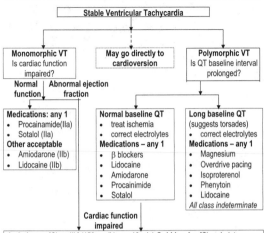

Stable Ventricular Tachycardia

Monomorphic VT
Is cardiac function impaired?

May go directly to cardioversion

Polymorphic VT
Is QT baseline interval prolonged?

Normal function | Abnormal ejection fraction

Medications: any 1
- Procainamide(IIa)
- Sotalol (IIa)

Other acceptable
- Amiodarone (IIb)
- Lidocaine (IIb)

Normal baseline QT
- treat ischemia
- correct electrolytes

Medications – any 1
- β blockers
- Lidocaine
- Amiodarone
- Procainimide
- Sotalol

Long baseline QT
(suggests torsades)
- correct electrolytes

Medications – any 1
- Magnesium
- Overdrive pacing
- Isoproterenol
- Phenytoin
- Lidocaine

All class indeterminate

Cardiac function impaired

Amiodarone [Class IIb] (150 mg IV over 10 min) **Or Lidocaine** [Class Indeterminate] (0.5-0.75 mg/kg IV push). Then **Synchronized cardioversion** see below
See pages 30-34 for drug dosing.

Tachycardia - Synchronized Cardioversion Algorithm –for tachycardia with serious signs/symptoms related to tachycardia (not for pulseless VT or VF)

If ventricular rate is > 150 (generally not needed ≤ 150), prepare for immediate cardioversion. May give brief trial of medications based on specific arrhythmia.

⇩

Have at bedside (1) O_2 sat monitor, (2) suction, (3) IV, (4) intubation equipment, then premedicate when appropriate (e.g. midazolam, propofol, methohexital)

⇩

Synchronized Cardioversion

- **Rhythms** - VT, SVT, atrial fibrillation and flutter
- **Energy levels**– 100J, 200J, 300J, 360 J monophasic energy dose or equivalent biphasic (exception, SVT and atrial flutter – start with 50 joules)
- **If delays** in synchronization & critically ill, go straight to unsynchronized mode

Myocardial Infarction (MI) & Acute Coronary Syndromes (ACS)

Utility of Various Tests for Diagnosis of Acute MI/ Cardiac Ischemia

Table below details predictive values for diagnosis of Acute Myocardial Infarction if non-italicized and *Acute Cardiac Ischemia (ACI)* if italicized.

Diagnostic Test	Sensitivity	Specificity	PPV[k]	NPV[k]
12 lead ECG (liberal criteria)[a]	94-99	19-27	21	98
12 lead ECG (intermediate criteria)[b]	69-75	83-86	44	95
12 lead ECG (strict criteria)[c]	38-44	97-98	76	91
15 lead ECG (+V8,V9,V4R)	55-60[h]	97-98		
22 lead ECG (many AP thorax leads)	88[h]	---		
Continuous/serial ECG (ACI)	*21-25*	*92-99*		
Continuous/serial ECG	39	88		
ECG stress test (ACI)	*68[i]*	*77*		
CK-MB enzymes over 24 h	100	98		
CK-MB serial (ACI)	*31*	*95*		Data sources:
1st CK-MB, pain onset < 4 h prior	41	88		(1)*Ann Emerg*
1st CK-MB, pain onset > 4 h prior	63	90		*Med 2001; 37:*
Serial CK-MB isoform, pain = 4 h[d]	56	93		*453.*
Serial CK-MB isoform, pain = 6 h[d]	96	94		(2) *Ann Emerg*
CK-MB at 0,1,2,3 h after ED arrival[e]	80	94		*Med 1997; 29(1)*
Myoglobin, pain onset = 2 h prior	89	96		(3) *Acad Emerg*
Myoglobin, pain onset 12-24 h prior	59	95		*Med 1997;4:13.*
P-selectin	45	76		(4) *Ann Emerg*
Troponin T, pain onset = 2 h prior	33	100		*Med 1992; 21:*
Troponin T, pain onset = 6 h prior	78	99		*504*
Troponin T, pain onset 12-24 h prior	93	99		
Rest echocardiography[f]	81-91	43-83		
Rest echocardiography (ACI)	*43-88*	*72-94*		
Stress echocardiography	90	89		
Sestamibi rest (technetium 99m scan)[g]	*74-87*	*56-85*		
Sestamibi rest (ACI)	*78-98*	*52-79*		

[a] nonspecific ST segment or T wave changes abnormal but not diagnostic of ischemia; Or ischemia, strain, or infarction known or not known to be old.

[b] ST segment ↑↓, or T wave changes consistent with ischemia/strain, not known to be old.

[c] ST segment elevation or pathologic Q waves not known to be old.

[d] CK-MB isoforms were collected every 30-60 minutes for at least 6 hours after symptom onset when studied. Criteria for AMI diagnosis: MB2 > 1U/L or MB2/MB1 > 1.5.

[e] Sensitivity/specificity if > 6 hours from pain onset. Numbers are lower if < 6 hours.

[f] Sensitivity/specificity if obtained during chest pain.

[g] Must have ongoing chest pain and no nitrate or β blocker administered before test.

[h] Sensitivity using criteria strict ECG above

[i] Sensitivity is higher for three vessel disease and lower if LVH noted on ECG.

[j] NPV - negative predictive value, PPV - positive predictive value

Acute Chest Pain/Coronary Syndrome Algorithm

Immediate Assessment	Immediate General Treatment[1]
• Vital, O_2 saturation, IV access, ECG • Exam & fibrinolytic eligibility < 10 min • Obtain serum cardiac markers, CXR, electrolytes, coagulation studies	• Oxygen, Aspirin 160-325 mg PO • Nitroglycerin SL or spray q 5 min X 3 • Morphine IV titrate to pain (if pain not relieved by nitroglycerin)

Assess initial ECG within 10 minutes of ED arrival

ST elevation, new or presumably new LBBB	ST depression, dynamic T wave invert with pain	Nondiagnostic ECG no ST-T wave changes
• ST elevation ≥ 1 mm In ≥ 2 contiguous leads, • New/presumably new LBBB (obscuring ST segment analysis)	•ST depression > 1 mm •Marked symmetrical T wave inversion multiple precordial leads •Dynamic ST-T changes	•ST depression ½-1 mm •T-wave inverted/flat in leads with dominant R •Normal ECG
• > 90% with ischemia and ST elevation will develop new Q or ⊕ serum markers for MI • Patients with hyper-acute T waves when acute MI certain • ST depressed in early precordial leads with posterior MI	**High risk patient with increased mortality** • Persistent symptoms • Recurrent ischemia • Poor LV function • Widespread ECG Δ • Congestive failure • ⊕ cardiac markers • old MI, CABG, stent or angioplasty	**Heterogeneous group Rapid assessment** • Serial ECGs • ST segment monitoring • Cardiac markers **Further assessment helpful** • Perfusion radionuclide scanning • Stress echo
• Aspirin 160-325 mg • β-blocker IV • Nitroglycerin IV • Heparin if fibrin specific lytics • Thrombolytics[2] Or Angioplasty/stent	• Aspirin 160-325 mg • β-blocker IV • Nitroglycerin IV • Heparin IV • Glycoprotein IIb/IIIa inhibitors[3] • ±PCI [2]	• Aspirin 160-325 mg • Other therapy as appropriate for etiology • If ⊕ serum markers ECG changes, or functional study manage as High risk above

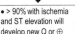

[1] Substitute clopidogrel if unable to take aspirin (withhold for 5-7 days pre CABG).

[2] See page 30-36 for specific medication, thrombolytic dosing, and PCI recommendations.

[3] Abciximab (*Reopro*), Eptifibatide (*Integrilin*), Tirofiban (*Aggrastat*)

Circulation 2000; 102: I 178;   2002; 106: 1893.

Indications for Transcutaneous Patches/Pacing in Acute MI

Hemodynamically unstable bradycardia (< 50 bpm)

Mobitz type II 2nd degree AV block, or 3rd degree heart block

Bilateral BBB, Alternating BBB or RBBB and alternating LBBB

Left anterior fascicular block or newly acquired or age-indeterminate LBBB

RBBB or LBBB and 1st degree AV block

Circulation 2000: 102: (suppl).

American Heart Association/American College of Cardiology Guidelines for Ambulatory Electrocardiography (AECG).

	To Assess Symptoms Possibly Related to Rhythm Disturbance
Class I	• Syncope, near syncope, or episodic dizziness without obvious cause • Unexplained recurrent palpitations
Class IIb	• Episodic shortness of breath, chest pain, or fatigue without cause • Neurologic symptoms if transient atrial fibrillation/flutter is suspected • Syncope, near syncope, episodic dizziness, or palpitations when other causes are identified, but symptoms persist
Class III	• Syncope, near syncope, episodic dizziness, or palpitations when other cause is identified • Cerebrovascular accidents without other evidence or arrhythmia
	To Assess Patients Without Symptoms of Arrhythmia
Class I	• None
Class IIb	• Post-MI with LV dysfunction, CHF or IHSS
Class III	• Myocardial contusion, systemic hypertension, with LV hypertrophy • Post-MI with normal LV function • Preoperative arrhythmia evaluation for noncardiac surgery • Sleep apnea or valvular heart disease

ACC/AHA. *J Am Coll Cardiol* 1999; 34: 913.

Select Parenteral Cardiovascular Medications & AHA/ACC Guidelines
[*Circulation* 2000; 102:1193; 2002; 106: 1896] (www.americanheart.org)

Abciximab (Reopro)	• PCI – 0.25 mg/kg IV pre PCI, + 0.125 µg/kg/min (maximum of 10 µg/min) X 12 h after PCI **Class I** – *UA/NSTEMI* –for 12-24 hours if PCI planned next 24 hours **Class III** – *UA/NSTEMI* – patients in whom PCI is not planned
ACE inhibitors	**Class I** – (1) 1st 24 hours of acute MI with ST elevation in > 2 anterior precordial leads or CHF without ↓ BP or contraindication (2) UA/NSTEMI –hypertension despite treatment with NTG & β blocker if LV systolic dysfunction or CHF and in patients with diabetes. **Class IIa** – all other within 24 h of suspected MI. All post acute coronary syndrome patients. **Class IIb** – after recovery from MI with normal or mildly abnormal left ventricular function.
Adenosine (Adenocard)	• SVT – 6 mg IV. Repeat 12 mg IV q 2 min X 2 doses. Avoid if: 2nd/3rd degree AV block, sick sinus syndrome, on dipyridamole
Alteplase (t-PA)	• See thrombolytics page 36
Amiodarone (Cordarone)	• VF/pulseless VT – 300 mg IVP • Recurrent VF/Pulseless VT – 150 mg IVP • Ventricular arrhythmias – 150 mg IV over 10 minutes, then 1 mg/min X 6 h (360 mg), then 0.5 mg/min X 18 h (540 mg) **Class IIa** – (1) monomorphic VT with normal cardiac function (2) Atrial fibrillation/flutter with normal cardiac function **Class IIb** – (1) VF/pulseless VT (2) monomorphic VT with impaired cardiac function (3) polymorphic VT (4)Atrial fibrillation/flutter-impaired cardiac function/underlying WPW
Argatroban (formerly Acova) Use if heparin induced thrombo-cytopenia	• UA/NSTEMI/Pre-PCI – 350 µg/kg IV over 3-5 minutes plus 25 µg/kg/min. Check activated clotting time (ACT) 5-10 min. after bolus complete. Therapeutic ACT is 300-450 sec. If ACT < 300 sec., administer 2nd bolus of 150 µg/kg and ↑ infusion to 30 µg/kg/min and recheck ACT in 5-10 minutes. If ACT > 450 sec., ↓ infusion to 15 µg/kg/min and recheck ACT in 5-10 minutes. May take with aspirin.
Aspirin	• Acute MI – 160 – 325 mg PO **Class I** – *MI/UA/NSTEMI* – begin immediately **Class IIb** - If allergy, choose clopidogrel over ticlopidine, dipyridamole
Atenolol (Tenormin)	• Acute MI – 5 mg IV over 5 minutes, repeat in 10 minutes, then 50 mg/day increased to 50 mg BID as tolerated. **Class I** – *MI/UA/NSTEMI* – Within 12 hr of MI or ongoing, recurrent pain. **Class IIb** – *Acute MI* –moderate LV failure (bibasilar rales without low cardiac output) or other relative contraindications to β blockers, provided patients can be monitored closely. **Class III** *MI/UA/NSTEMI* – severe LV failure, ↓ HR, contraindications

Class I - treatment is beneficial, useful, & effective.; *Class IIa* - evidence favors efficacy. (IIb) - efficacy less well established.; *Class III* may be harmful, usually contraindicated. [1-4] PCI – procedural coronary intervention, MI – myocardial infarction, UA – unstable angina, NSTEMI – nonST elevation MI

Atropine	• <u>Asystole</u> – 1 mg IV, repeat q 3-5 minutes (Max 0.04 mg/kg) • <u>Bradycardia</u> 0.5 – 1.0 mg IV q 3-5 minutes (Max 0.04 mg/kg) ET dose is 2-3 mg diluted in 10 ml NS. ***Class I – Acute MI** – (1) sinus bradycardia with low cardiac output & hypoperfusion, or frequent PVCs at onset of acute MI (2) inferior MI with type I 2nd or 3rd AV block & ↓BP, ischemic pain or ventricular arrhythmias (3) sustained ↓ HR/BP after nitroglycerin (4) nausea and vomiting associated with morphine (5) asystole* ***Class IIa – Acute MI** – symptomatic inferior infarction and type I 2nd or 3rd degree heart block at AV node (narrow QRS or known BBB)* ***Class IIb- Acute MI** – (1) administration with morphine in the presence of bradycardia (2) asymptomatic with inferior infarction and type I 2nd or 3rd degree heart block at the AV node (3) 2nd or 3rd degree AV block of uncertain mechanism when pacing unavailable* ***Class III – Acute MI** – sinus bradycardia > 40 without hypoperfusion or frequent PVCs (2) type II AV block or 3rd degree AV block with new wide QRS complex presumed due to MI*
Bivalirudin (Angiomax)	• Indication: a direct thrombin inhibitor used if unstable angina and undergoing PCI (if heparin allergy/thrombocytopenia) • 1 mg/kg IV bolus prior to PCI, then 2.5 mg/kg/hour for 4 hours. Additional infusion of 0.2 mg/kg/hour may be continued for another 20 hours. Use with aspirin.
Bumetanide	• (Bumex) 0.5-1.0 mg IV/IM; 1mg *Bumex* ~ 40 mg *Lasix*
Clopidogrel (Plavix)	• 300 mg PO loading dose, then 75 mg PO q day ***Class I – UA/NSTEMI** – (1) all patients unable to take aspirin (2) add to aspirin in all not requiring procedural intervention (withhold 5-7 days if elective CABG is planned). Withhold for 5-7 days if elective CABG planned. Otherwise continue for 1-9 months.*
Dalteparin	• UA/NSTEMI – 120 units/kg SC q 12 h. Max dose 10,000 units
Digoxin (Lanoxin)	• Rapid Afib - 0.25 mg IV q 2 hours up to 1.5 mg. ***Class Ib – Afib** - if congestive heart failure* ***Class IIb – Afib** - rate control if no congestive heart failure*
Diltiazem (Cardizem)	• 20 mg (0.25 mg/kg) IV over 2 min. Repeat 25 mg (0.35 mg/kg) IV 15 min after 1st dose prn. Drip at 5-15 mg/h prn ***Class I – UANSTEMI** –continuing or recurring ischemia when β blockers are contraindicated & no contraindications. **Class I – Atrial Fib/flutte/SVT**– preserved LV function – rate control **Class IIa– UANSTEMI** – oral long acting agents if recurrent ischemia in absence of contraindications & β blockers/nitrates are fully used. **Class IIb – Atrial Fib/flutter** – if CHF; **Class IIb– UANSTEMI** – (1) extended release form of nondihydro-pyridine calcium antagonist (diltiazem, verapamil) instead of β blocker Or (2) immediate release dihydropyridine calcium antagonist (nifedipine) in presence of a β blocker. **Class III** – Atrial fibrillation/flutter – if preexcitation - WPW*

Class I   - treatment is beneficial, useful, & effective.; *Class IIa* - evidence favors efficacy. *(IIb)* - efficacy less well established.; *Class III* may be harmful, usually contraindicated
[1-4] PCI – procedural coronary intervention, MI – myocardial infarction, UA – unstable angina, NSTEMI – nonST elevation MI

Dobutamine (*Dobutrex*)	• 2-20 µg/kg/min IV; 250 mg in 250 ml NS or D5W = 1 mg/ml
Dopamine (*Intropin*)	• 2-50 µg/kg/min IV, Mix 400 mg in 250 ml D5W = 1.6 mg/ml. • 1-5 µg/kg/min (renal), 5-10 µg/kg/min (cardiac), > 10 µg/kg/min (vasoconstriction), > 40 consider norepinephrine
Enoxaparin (*Lovenox*)	• UA/NSTEMI/PCI – 1 mg/kg SC q 12 hours (with aspirin) and continued ≥ 2 days until clinically stable. Maximum single dose is 150 mg SC. OD associated with severe bleeding may be reversed by slow infusion of protamine sulfate IV. See heparin below for specific AHA/ACC recommendations
Epinephrine (*Adrenalin*)	• <u>Cardiac arrest</u> – 1.0 mg IV q 3-5 min. (10 ml of 1:10,000 followed by 20 ml NS flush). ET dose: 2-2.5 mg • <u>Shock</u> – 2 –10 µg/min. IV infusion. Mix 1 mg in 500 ml NS and infuse at 1-5 ml/min. *Class Indeterminate – use in cardiac arrest*
Eptifibatide (*Integrelin*)	• PCI – 135 µg/kg IV, plus 0.5 µg/kg/min X 20-24 hours • UA/NSTEMI – 180 µg/kg IV, + 2 µg/kg/min X 72-96 h. If serum creatinine > 2 mg/dl or creatinine clearance < 50 ml/min bolus with same amount and decrease infusion rate to 1 µg/kg/min. *Class I – UA/NSTEMI – PCI is planned and heparin/aspirin are given* *Class IIa – UA/NSTEMI – (1) in addition to aspirin and heparin if ongoing chest pain or ⊕ cardiac markers or other high risk features when PCI and catheterization not planned (2) if already receiving heparin, aspirin, and clopidogrel when PCI or catheterization is planned. Class IIb – UA/NSTEMI – (1) patients without continuing ischemia with no other high risk features and PCI is not planned*
Esmolol (*Brevibloc*)	• SVT/AF/Flutter/(Torsades with normal baseline QT) – Load 500µg/kg IV over 1 min, then 50 µg/kg/min X 4 min. If no response, 500 µg/kg IV over 1 min, then 100 µg/kg/min X 4 min. Continue to repeat 500 µg/kg over 1 min prn while increasing infusion by 50 µg/kg/min until desired effect achieved or max. of 300 µg/kg/min. Once adequate response, do not change rate > 25 µg/kg/min or rebolus. *Class I – Afib – rate control*
Furosemide	• (*Lasix*) 0.5-2.0 mg/kg IV
Group IIb/IIIa	(Inhibitors) – see Abciximab, Eptifibatide and Tirofiban
Heparin or Low Molecular Weight Heparin (LMWH) – Enoxaparin Lovenox	• UA/NSTEMI/PCI – 80 U/kg IV + 18 U/kg/h, titrate to PTT • MI/alteplase use – 60 U/kg IV (max 4,000 U), + 12 U/kg/h [max 1000 U/h] (PTT goal 50-70 sec or 1.5-2.0 X control) *Class I –UA/NSTEMI – add to aspirin and or clopidogrel* *Class IIa – (1) Lovenox is preferred over unfractionated heparin in UA/NSTEMI in absence of renal failure unless CABG planned in 24 hours. (2) MI – IV X 48 h if tPA given, if high risk for emboli (large/anterior MI, atrial fibrillation, prior embolus, known LV clot) IV unfractionated heparin preferred Class IIb – SC use if nonselective thrombolytics administered and low risk for emboli until ambulatory* • In patients at risk for heparin induced thrombocytopenia, argatroban may be substituted. (See argatroban page 30)

Isoproterenol *(Isuprel)*	• <u>Bradycardia</u> – 2 – 10 µg/min IV (if atropine, dopamine have failed and no pacer available) ***Class indeterminate*** – polymorphic VT as temporizing measure
Lidocaine	• <u>Vfib/Pulseless Vtach</u> - 1.0-1.5 mg/kg IV (2-4 mg/kg ET) may repeat 0.5-0.75 mg/kg IV over 3-5 minutes (Max 3 mg/kg) • <u>Vtach – monomorphic</u>, stable, normal cardiac function 1.0-1.5 mg/kg IV q 5-10 min.; <u>Vtach – impaired cardiac function</u> – 0.5 – 0.75 mg/kg IV q 5-10 minutes. (Max 3 mg/kg) • If conversion with lidocaine infuse 1-4 mg/min IV ***Class IIa*** – for 24-48 hours after ventricular fibrillation/tachycardia ***Class IIb***– sustained monomorphic ventricular tachycardia (VT) not associated with angina hypotension or CHF. ***Class III*** – prophylaxis with thrombolytics, isolated PVC's, couplets, accelerated idioventricular rhythm, nonsustained VT ***Class Indeterminate*** – pulseless Vfib/Vtach, (2) monomorphic ventricular tachycardia with impaired cardiac function.
Magnesium	• <u>Torsades/Various tachyarrhythmias</u> – 2 g IV over 15 minutes ***Class I*** – no class I recommendations ***Class IIa*** – Treating ↓K, ↓Mg, or torsades de pointes (indeterminate)
Metoprolol *(Lopressor)*	• <u>Acute MI</u> – 5 mg IV q 5 min X 3, then 50 mg PO q 12 h X 24 hours, then ↑ to 100 mg q 12 h or 50 mg q 6 h as tolerated • Afib- 2.5-5.0 mg IV (over 2 min) q 5 min, up to 3 doses ***Class I – MI/UA/NSTEMI*** - <12 h of MI with ongoing, recurrent pain ***Class I – Afib*** – if no congestive heart failure ***Class IIb – Afib*** – if congestive heart failure ***Class III*** – heart failure, bradycardia or other contraindication
Nitroglycerin	• <u>MI/CHF/UA/NSTEMI</u> – Initiate at 10-20 µg/min IV. Increase 5-20 µg/min q 3-5 min until desired effect. ***Class I*** – (1) 1st 24 – 48 hours in acute MI with CHF, large anterior infarct, persistent ischemia or hypertension. (2) continued use (> 48 h) if recurrent angina, or persistent pulmonary congestion. ***Class IIb*** – (1) 1st 24-48 hours after MI without ↓ BP, ↑HR or ↓HR (2) continued use (> 48 h) if large or complicated infarction ***Class III*** – systolic BP < 90 mm Hg or heart rate < 50/minue, Or within 24 hours of sildenafil (Viagra) use
Norepinephrine *(Levophed)*	• <u>Shock</u> – 0.5-1 µg/min, ↑1-2 µg/min q 3-5 min until desired effect. Usual maintenance dose is 2-4 µg/min, occasionally 8-30 µg/min is required. Use central line if possible.
Oxygen	***Class I*** (1) overt pulmonary congestion, (2) O_2 saturation < 90% ***Class IIa*** – routine to all uncomplicated MIs in 1st 2-3 hours. ***Class III*** - routine to all uncomplicated MIs > 3-6 hours.

Class I - treatment is beneficial, useful, & effective.; *Class IIa* - evidence favors efficacy. *(IIb)* - efficacy less well established.; *Class III* may be harmful, usually contraindicated. [1-4] PCI – procedural coronary intervention, MI – myocardial infarction, UA – unstable angina, NSTEMI – nonST elevation MI

Procainamide	• <u>Afib/Flutter,Wide complex tachycardia</u> - 20 mg/min IV (max total dose 17 mg/kg) until (1) ↓BP, (2) QRS complex increases 50%, (3) arrhythmia stops or (4) total 17 mg/kg • <u>VF/pulseless VT</u> –50 mg/min IV (up to max dose 17 mg/min) *Class IIa* - stable SVT/Atrial fib/flutter/ventricular tachycardia. *Class IIb* – polymorphic VT, or SVT in WPW
Protamine sulfate	• 1 mg protamine neutralizes 100 units unfractionated heparin, 100 anti-Xa units of dalteparin or tinzaparin, OR 1 mg of enoxaparin (*Lovenox*). If aPTT is still elevated 2-4 hours after initial protamine dose, give 0.5 mg protamine for each 100 anti-Xa units of dalteparin or tinzaparin OR each 1 mg of enoxaparin. Administer by slow IV injection of 1% solution over > 10 minutes. Maximum dose is 50 mg. • Observe for anaphylaxis/hypotension if given too rapidly. Increased risk of allergic reaction if prior exposure (e.g. insulin), fish allergy, vasectomy (anti-protamine antibodies) . • Protamine reverses anti-thrombin activity but only partially reverses anti-Xa activity.
Reteplase	(*Retavase*) see thrombolytics page 36
Sodium Nitroprusside	• 0.1 µg/kg/min IV titrated up q 3-5 minutes to desired effect up to maximum of 5 µg/kg/min
Streptokinase	(*Streptase*) see thrombolytics page 36
Tenecteplase	(*TNKase*) see thrombolytics page 36
Thrombolytics	• See page 36
Tirofiban (*Aggrastat*)	• <u>UA/NTESMI/PCI</u> – 0.4 µg/kg/min X 30 min, then 0.1 µg/kg/min X 48-108 hours or until 24 hours after procedure. *Class I – UA/NSTEMI - PCI is planned and heparin/aspirin are given* *Class IIa – UA/NSTEMI – (1) in addition to aspirin and heparin if ongoing chest pain or ⊕ cardiac markers or other high risk features if PCI and catheterization not planned (2) patients already receiving heparin, aspirin, and clopidogrel & PCI or catheterization is planned* *Class IIb – UA/NSTEMI – (1) patients without continuing ischemia who have no other high risk features and in whom PCI is not planned*
Vasopressin	• <u>Vfib/Pulseless Vtach</u> – 40 units IV. No repeat dose. • <u>Asystole</u> – 40 units IV q 3 min X 2. May follow with epi prn.
Verapamil (*Calan*)	• <u>SVT</u> – 2.5-5.0 mg IV over 2 minutes. May repeat 5-10 mg IV over 2 minutes, 15-30 minutes after 1st dose • <u>Afib</u> – 0.075 – 0.15 mg/kg IV over 2 min. *Class I – Afib – no congestive heart failure* *Class IIb – Afib – congestive heart failure*

Class I - treatment is beneficial, useful, & effective.; *Class IIa* - evidence favors efficacy.
(IIb) - efficacy less well established.; *Class III* may be harmful, usually contraindicated
[1-4] PCI – procedural coronary intervention, MI – myocardial infarction, UA – unstable angina, NSTEMI – nonST elevation MI

AHA/ACC Guidelines for Specific Cardiac Procedures[1-4]

Angiography If no primary PCI (see PCI – below)	**Class I - Acute MI** – none unless PCI **Class IIa - Acute MI** – cardiogenic shock/hemodynamically unstable **Class IIb - Acute MI** –evolving large or anterior infarct treated with thrombolytics (without effect) and adjuvant PTCA is planned. **Class III - Acute MI** – routine angiography/PCI ≤ 24 h of thrombolytic
Intra-aortic balloon pump	**Class II a - UA/NSTEMI** – severe ischemia that is continuing or recurs frequently despite intensive medical therapy or for hemodynamic instability in patients before or after coronary angiography
Procedural Coronary Intervention (PCI)	**Class I - Acute MI** – (1) alternative to thrombolytics if Acute MI and ST elevation or new/presumed new LBBB who can undergo angioplasty of the infarct artery within 12 h of symptom onset or beyond 12 h if ischemic symptoms persist; if performed in a timely fashion (90 ± 30 minutes of admission) if skilled (> 75 procedures/y) in an appropriate environment (center with > 200 procedures/y), (2) within 36 h of an acute ST elevation/Q wave or new LBBB MI with cardiogenic shock age < 75 years old and revascularization can be performed within 18 h of onset of shock **Class I - UA/NSTEMI** – early invasive strategy if UA/NSTEMI and no serious comorbordity if any of (1) recurrent angina/ischemia at rest or with low level activity despite therapy (2) elevated troponin (3) new or presumably ST depression (4) recurrent angina/ischemia with CHF, an S3, pulmonary edema, worsening rales, or worsening mitral regurgitation (5) high risk noninvasive stress test (6) EF < 40%, (7) hemodynamic instability (h) sustained ventricular tachycardia (8) PCI in prior 6 months (9) prior CABG. **Class IIa - Acute MI** –reperfusion if contraindication to thrombolytics **Class IIa - UA/NSTEMI** - focal saphenous vein graft lesions or multiple stenoses in poor candidates for reoperative surgery. **Class IIb - Acute MI** –acute MI without ST elevation but with reduced (< TIMI grade 2) flow of the infarct related artery and when angioplasty can be performed within 12 hours of onset of symptoms. **Class IIb- UA/NSTEMI** - 2 or 3 vessel disease with significant proximal LAD CAD with treated diabetes or abnormal LV function and with anatomy suitable for catheter based therapy. **Class III - Acute MI** – (1) elective angioplasty of non infarct artery at time of MI, (2) > 12 h post symptoms and no acute MI, (3) post-fibrinolytic therapy and no ischemic symptoms (4) are eligible for thrombolysis & primary angioplasty performed by a low volume operator in a lab without surgical capability **Class III - UA/NSTEMI** - 1 or 2 vessel CAD without significant proximal LAD CAD or with mild symptoms or unlikely due to ischemia or who have not received adequate medical therapy and have no ischemia on noninvasive testing. (2) insignificant coronary stenosis (< 50%) (3) significant left main CAD who are candidates for CABG

Class I - treatment is beneficial, useful, & effective.; *Class IIa* - evidence favors efficacy. *(IIb)* - efficacy less well established.; *Class III* may be harmful, usually contraindicated
[1-4] PCI – procedural coronary intervention, MI – myocardial infarction, UA – unstable angina, NSTEMI – nonST elevation MI

AHA/ACC Recommendations for Thrombolytic Therapy in Acute MI

Class	Recommendation
I	• ST elevation > 0.1 mV in ≥ 2 contiguous leads **AND** time to therapy of ≤ 12 hours **AND** age < 75 years • New bundle branch block **AND** history highly suggestive of acute MI
II a	• ST elevation > 0.1 mV in ≥ 2 contiguous leads **AND** age ≥ 75 years
II b	• ST elevation > 0.1 mV in ≥ 2 contiguous leads + time to therapy 12-24 h • Presenting systolic BP > 180 mm Hg or diastolic BP > 110 mm Hg with **high-risk MI**. An attempt to lower BP 1st with β blockers, or nitrates is recommended but not proven to lower risk of intracranial hemorrhage. **High risk MI** – female, age > 70 years, prior MI, atrial fibrillation, anterior MI, rales in > 1/3 of lung fields, low BP, sinus tachycardia or diabetes
III	• ST elevation + time to therapy > 24 h **Or** ST segment depression only

Class I - treatment is beneficial, useful, & effective.; _Class IIa_ - evidence favors efficacy.
Class IIb- efficacy less well established.; _Class III_ - treatment not useful, may be harmful,
usually contraindicated

J Am Coll Cardiol 1996; 28: 1328.

Absolute Contraindications to Thrombolytic Use

Prior CNS bleed or CNS neoplasm	Active internal bleeding (not menses)
Stroke/TIA in past 1 year	Suspect aortic dissection, pericarditis

Relative Contraindications or Cautions to Thrombolytic Use

BP > 180/110 (arrival or during treatment)	Noncompressible vascular puncture
Anticoagulation (INR ≥ 2), bleed diathesis	Internal bleeding in past 2-4 weeks
Ready high volume cardiac cath. lab	Streptokinase use (1-2 years), tPA is OK
History or prior stroke or known CNS pathology not included above	Recent trauma (<2-4 weeks) (head/spine trauma, CPR > 10 min, major surgery)
Pregnancy, active peptic ulcer	History of chronic severe hypertension

J Am Coll Cardiol 1996; 28: 1328.

Thrombolytic Dose and Choice of Agent

Agent[1]	Dose	Criteria
r-PA	• 10 U IV over 2 min, repeat dose in 30 min • Administer heparin as detailed for tPA	• See tPA below
TNK-ase	• Single IV bolus over 5 seconds; if < 60 kg (30 mg), 60-69 kg (35 mg), 70-79 kg (40 mg), 80-89 kg (45 mg), ≥ 90 kg (50 mg)	• See tPA below
t-PA	• 15 mg bolus + 0.75 mg/kg (max 50 mg) over 30 min + 0.50 mg/kg (max. 35 mg) over 60 min + heparin 60 U/kg bolus + 12 U/kg/h. PTT goal is 1.5-2.0 X control.	• Age ≤ 75 years • Anterior Wall or _possibly_ large inferior-lateral MI derive most benefit
SK	• 1.5 million U. IV over 1 hour	• All others (unless prior SK)

r-PA – reteplase (_Retavase_); t-PA – tissue plasminogen activator or alteplase (_Activase_); SK –
streptokinase (_Streptase_), tenecteplase (_TNKase_)

North American Society Pacing & Electrophysiology Generic Pacemaker Code

I Chamber Paced	II Chamber Sensed	III Response to sensing	IV Programmability, rate modulation	V Antitachy-dysrhythmia functions
O – None	O – None	O – None	O – None	O – None
A – Atrium	A – Atrium	T – Triggered	P– Simple programmable	P – Pacing Anti dysrhythmia
V – Ventricle	V – Ventricle	I – Inhibited	M– multiprogrammable	S– shock
D – Dual (A and V)	D – Dual (A and V)	D – Dual (A triggered & A + V inhibited)	C – Communicating	D – dual pacing and shock

Pacemaker Malfunction Evaluation & Management

Evaluate EKG without and with magnet. Right ventricular leads typically cause left bundle/left axis appearance to paced rhythm. New right bundle suggests septal perforation. In most (not all) pacemakers, magnet eliminates sensing and causes asynchronous pacing (e.g. AOO, VOO, DOO).

Problem	Recognition & Management
Battery old	May cause gradual slowing of paced rate, or sensing stops and asynchronous pacing. Failure to pace/capture can occur.
Defibrillation	If electrical cardioversion or defibrillation is required, place paddles as far from the pulse generator as possible. Also, place paddles perpendicular to the axis of the pacemaker generator and electrodes (usually anteroposterior placement). Have external pacemaker ready after any cardioversion/defibrillation.
Failure to pace (Output failure)	This occurs when a pacemaker does not deliver a stimulus to the heart. Patients may develop ↓ cardiac output (chest pain, shortness of breath, lightheaded, syncope) due to pacer pauses (esp. if patient pacer dependent). Atrial, ventricular (or both) pacer spikes normally seen on EKG may be absent. Causes (1) Oversensing: pacer senses skeletal muscle contraction or other form of electric interference (e.g. normal QRS complex, MRI, or cellular phone). Muscular interference can be reproduced by having patient tense pectoral or abdominal muscles. Short term can treat oversensing by turning on asynchronous mode via magnet. Other causes of oversensing include (2) lead fracture, dislodgement, disconnection (CXR can reveal these abnormalities sometimes) and (3) component failure (e.g. battery). Pseudomalfunction occurs if pacing artifacts in bipolar systems are present but not visible on EKG or when artifacts are absent due to appropriate inhibition of pacer when spontaneous rate is above the programmed threshold.

Pacemaker Malfunction Evaluation & Management - continued

Failure to capture	Pacer delivers stimulus (pacing artifact seen) & no myocardial depolarization occurs. Causes include lead displacement or fracture, battery depletion, elevated pacing threshold of myocardium (due to MI, electrolyte disturbance, meds [esp. IC anti-arrhythmics], external defibrillation), or prolonged myocardial refractoriness (e.g. prolonged QT syndrome). Treat underlying cause. IV isoproterenol may be effective in treating failure to capture due to high antiarrhythmic drug levels.
MRI use	Presence of a pacemaker is a contraindication to MRI study. However, programming pacemaker to an asynchronous mode before imaging can prevent injury from MRI.
Pacemaker mediated tachycardia	Reentry tachycardia in dual chamber pacers with atrial sensing and pacemaker acting as part of reentry circuit. Rate is variable but cannot rise above programmed upper limit of pacer. Application of magnet stops circuit and treats. Adenosine, carotid massage, and external pacer (pulse width of 40 msec) may end this tachycardia if rhythm is refractory to magnet application.
Pacemaker syndrome	Suboptimal pacing modes or programming leading to inadequate pacing with suboptimal AV synchrony (esp. VVI or VVO pacers) or AV dyssynchrony (with increased atrial pressure, cannon A waves etc) leading to no atrial kick to cardiac output (lower cardiac output/BP, syncope, shortness of breath, fatigue), mitral regurgitation, or tricuspid insufficiency. Systolic BP may drop > 20 mm Hg when spontaneous rhythm converted to a paced rhythm.
Runaway pacemaker	Inappropriate rapid discharges potentially leading to ventricular tachycardia or fibrillation. It is most commonly due to pacemaker component failure. Applying magnet may slow rate as well as emergency interrogation/reprogramming. Surgery may be needed to disconnect or cut leads.
Undersensing	Pacemaker fails to sense or detect native cardiac activity. EKG may be normal or may not respond to appropriate signals (e.g. DDD system showing P wave but no intrinsic or paced QRS). Causes - new bundle branch, MI, PVCs, ventricular or atrial arrhythmias, lead problems (disconnect, looseness, incorrect position), battery failure, defibrillation, program error (too high sensing thresholds). Treat by correcting underlying cause.

Pulmonary Edema, Hypotension, Cardiogenic Shock Management

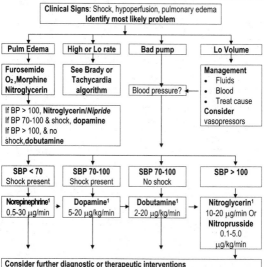

```
┌──────────────────────────────────────────────────────┐
│ Clinical Signs: Shock, hypoperfusion, pulmonary edema │
│          Identify most likely problem                 │
└──────────────────────────────────────────────────────┘
```

Pulm Edema	High or Lo rate	Bad pump	Lo Volume
Furosemide **O₂,Morphine** **Nitroglycerin**	See **Brady** or **Tachycardia** algorithm	Blood pressure?	**Management** • Fluids • Blood • Treat cause **Consider** vasopressors

If BP > 100, **Nitroglycerin**/*Nipride*
If BP 70-100 & shock, **dopamine**
If BP > 100, & no shock,**dobutamine**

SBP < 70 Shock present	SBP 70-100 Shock present	SBP 70-100 No shock	SBP > 100
Norepinephrine[1] 0.5-30 µg/min	**Dopamine**[1] 5-20 µg/kg/min	**Dobutamine**[1] 2-20 µg/kg/min	**Nitroglycerin**[1] 10-20 µg/min Or **Nitroprusside** 0.1-5.0 µg/kg/min

Consider further diagnostic or therapeutic interventions
Pulmonary artery catheter, Intra-aortic balloon pump, percutaneous coronary intervention for acute MI or ischemia, or other studies depending on situation.
[1]IV dose for all medications

CARDIAC PARAMETERS AND FORMULAS	Normal Values
Cardiac output (CO) = heart rate x stroke volume	4-8 L/min
Cardiac index (CI) = CO/BSA	2.8-4.2 L/min/m²
Mean arterial pressure (MAP) = (Systolic BP-Diastolic BP)/3 +Diastolic BP	80-100 mmHg
Systemic vascular resistance (SVR) = (MAP-CVP)(80)/CO	800-1200 dynes/sec/cm²
Pulmonary vascular resistance (PVR) = (PAM-PCWP)(80)/CO	45-120 dynes/sec/cm²
Central venous pressure (CVP)	5-12 cm H20
Pulmonary artery systolic pressure	20-30 mmHg
Pulmonary artery diastolic pressure	10-15 mmHg
Pulmonary artery mean pressure	15-20 mmHg
Pulmonary capillary wedge pressure (PCWP)	8-12 mmHg

Abdominal Aortic Aneurysm (AAA)

	Clinical Features of Ruptured AAA	

AAA-diameter ≥1.5X adjacent aorta or ≥ 3cm

Risk factors: male, family history (25% risk if AAA in sibling/parent), ↑ age, smoking, ↑BP peripheral or collagen vascular disease.

Radiologic evaluation: Plain films show calcified aortic wall in ~ 60%. Angiography can miss AAA with mural thrombus. US detects all AAA's but only leakage in 4%. CT identifies 100% of AAA's & > 95% rupture but not aorto-enteric or venous fistula, inflammatory aneurysms, or infections. Use MRI instead.

Clinical Features of Ruptured AAA	
Abdominal pain	77%
Flank or back pain	60%
Vomiting	25%
Syncope	18%
Hematemesis	5%
Known AAA	5%
Pulsatile mass	40-70%
Abdomen tenderness	41%
Pain, mass, and low BP	30-40%
Absent low ext. pulses	6%
Anuria or abd. bruit	< 1%

Management: (1) If rupture and unstable, resuscitate as needed, go to O.R. for repair (± bedside US). Do not delay repair. (2) If rupture and hemodynamically stable, cardiac monitor, O$_2$, large bore IV X 2 with NS. ECG, CXR, CBC, renal function, electrolytes & type and cross for ≥ 4-6 units of blood. Immediately notify surgeon. CT or MRI. *Emerg Med Reports* 1994; 15: 125.

Thoracic Aortic Dissection

	DeBakey Classification			
Classification of Thoracic Aortic Dissection	Type I - Ascending + descending aorta, Type II - Ascending aorta only, Type III - Distal to subclavian artery (IIIa above diaphragm and IIIb below diaphragm)			
	Stanford Classification			
	A – an ascending aorta involved, B – only descending aorta			

	Clinical Features	
	Chest or back pain	88%
	Aortic regurgitation ± congestive heart failure	50%
	Transitory pulse deficits	50%
Clinical Features	Neurologic deficits, hypotension (each 20%)	20%
	Syncope, tamponade, abdominal pain, GI bleed	variable
	hematuria, dyspnea, Horner's syndrome,	
	superior vena cava syndrome, and hemoptysis	

Diagnosis				
CXR Findings		**Diagnostic Study**	Sensitivity	Specificity
Any abnormality	85%	Transthoracic	-	-
Wide mediastinum	85%	echocardiography	75%	85-90%
Aortic knob abnormalities (Ca^{+2}	-	Angiography	85%	90-95%
separated > 5mm from knob a	-	Conventional CT	65-85%	95-100%
bulge or obliterated knob)	66%	Helical CT	90-100%	95-100%
Irregular aortic contour	38%	Transesophageal	-	-
Displaced trachea or NG tube	-	echocardiography	95-100%	90-97%
Left pleural effusion	27%	MRI	95-100%	95-100

J Emerg Med 1997; 15: 859; *Arch Intern Med* 2000; 160: 2977.; *Lancet* 1997; 349: 1461;

Thoracic Aortic Dissection - Management

If unstable, resuscitate & prepare for surgery. If stable, consult surgeon, control pain, BP & HR. Goal = HR of 60-80 & systolic BP = 90-110 mm Hg.

- Labetalol (*Normodyne*) - 0.25 mg/kg IV, double q 10 min up to 300 mg
- Alternately, use a β blocker + Nitroprusside. β blocker choices include (1, 2)
  1. propranolol (*Inderal*) 1-3 mg IV @ ≤ 1mg/min may repeat once in 5 minutes. Do not give additional doses in < 4 hours. **or**
  2. esmolol (*Brevibloc*) - bolus 500 µg/kg and start drip at 50-200 µg/kg/min
  3. sodium nitroprusside (*Nipride*) - 0.5 -10 µg/kg/min.
- Surgery is indicated for most ascending (Stanford A) dissections. Type B dissections are usually treated medically but occasionally require surgery.

Syncope

Syncope is a sudden temporary loss of consciousness with a loss of tone and spontaneous recovery. Relatively benign causes include vasodepressor syncope from excess vagal tone, micturation & defecation syncope, orthostatic syncope from dehydration or blood loss and drug induced syncope. Life threatening causes include dysrhythmias, aortic stenosis, MI, pulmonary embolus, vertebrobasilar transient ischemic attacks & cardiac conduction defects.

Cause of Syncope			
Cardiac 9-25%		**Not heart 34-46%**	
Vent tachycardia	11%	Orthostasis	10-21%
Sick sinus	3%	Vasovagal	8-9%
Complete heart		Situational	8%
or Mobitz II block	2%	Drugs	2-7%
SVT	2%	TIA	2-4%
Aortic stenosis	2%	Seizure	2-5%
MI, ↓HR	-	Others	1-8%
Carotid sinus	-	*Unknown 37-41%*	
Aortic dissection	1%	*NEJM 2002; 347:*	
Pulmonary	1%	*878.; Medicine*	
embolus		*1990; 69: 160*	

Diagnosis

Evaluation includes complete examination with rectal to look for occult blood, orthostatic vitals signs, a βhCG in women of child-bearing age, an ECG and pulse oximetry. Further evaluation is guided by the history and physical.

Studies Revealing Syncope Etiology	
History and physical exam	49%
Electrocardiographic monitoring	27%
Electrocardiogram	11%
Cardiac catheterization	7%
Electrophysiologic study	3%
Cerebral angiography	2%
Electroencephalography	1%

Management: If a cardiac or any life-threatening cause for syncope is likely, it must either be ruled out definitively in the emergency department or the patient must be admitted to the hospital (on continuous telemetry). The presence of an abnormal EKG (any abnormality except non-specific ST-T waves), CHF, prior ventricular arrhythmia, or age > 45 years denotes a 3 to 5 fold increased risk of cardiac disease causing syncope. These factors should increase the threshold for considering inpatient evaluation. If 3 out of 4 listed risk factors are present, mortality risk within one year is 58-80%. If no risk factors are present, 1 year mortality is 4-7%.

Ann Emerg Med 1997; 29: 459

Syncope continued...

San Francisco Syncope Rule	Criteria
The presence of any one or more of the bulleted features (**CHESS**) to the right was 96-98% sensitive and 58-62% specific in predicting serious disease, serious outcome, or deterioration within one week in ED patients in 2 studies.	• Congestive heart failure -Hx[1] • Hematocrit < 30% • EKG Abnormal[2] • Shortness of breath • Systolic BP (initial) < 90

[1] Hx – History of congestive heart failure, [2] New EKG changes or non-sinus rhythm.

Ann Emerg Med 2004; 43: 224; *Acad Emerg Med* 2004; 11: 529.

American College of Emergency Physicians Syncope Guidelines

Level	Specific Recommendations[1]
Level A	• <u>History</u>: no recommendations • <u>Examination</u>: no recommendations • <u>Testing</u>: no recommendations • <u>Admission</u>: no recommendations
Level B	• <u>History</u>: Age > 60 y + cardiovascular disease(CV) is high risk for adverse event. < 45 y & no CV disease or other risks is at low risk. • <u>Examination</u>: Congestive heart failure is high risk for adverse event. • <u>Testing</u>: Obtain an EKG if history/physical do not reveal a diagnosis. • <u>Admission</u>: Admit if history of congestive heart failure, ventricular arrhythmias, symptoms compatible with acute coronary syndrome, or evidence of CHF or valvular heart disease on examination, or EKG showing ischemia, prolonged QT interval, or bundle branch block.
Level C	• <u>History</u>: Reflex mediated or vasovagal syncope is a low risk for adverse events (AE). • <u>Examination</u>: Cardiac outflow obstruction is a high risk for AE. • <u>Testing</u>: Initiate cardiac monitoring if history and physical examination do not reveal diagnosis or cause of syncope. • <u>Admission</u>: Consider admission if age > 60 y, history of coronary artery disease or congenital heart disease, family history of unexplained sudden death, or exertional syncope in younger patients without an obvious etiology.

Level A – generally accepted principles of management.   www.acep.org

Level B – a range of strategies with moderate clinical certainty

Level C – strategies based on preliminary, inconclusive or conflicting evidence.

Valvular Heart Disease

Disorder	Murmur	Clinical features
Aortic regurgitation	high-pitched, blowing diastolic, after S2	dyspnea, fatigue, pulmonary edema, chest pain, wide pulse pressure
Aortic stenosis (AS)	harsh, systolic ejection right 2nd IC space to carotids, paradoxic S2 split, S3/S4 common	dyspnea (earliest symptom), syncope, angina, narrow pulse pressure, ECG with LVH, or (RBBB or LBBB in 10%)
Idiopathic Hypertrophic, Subaortic Stenosis (IHSS)	crescendo-decrescendo harsh systolic at apex or left sternal border.	similar to AS symptoms with earlier age onset (30-40 years), louder with exercise, and softer with squatting
Mitral regurgitation (Acute)	harsh apical systolic, crescendo-decrescendo starts at S1 + ends before S2, S3+S4	dyspnea, tachycardia, and acute pulmonary edema, angina (may be masked by dyspnea), shock. ECG without left atrial or vent. hypertrophy
Mitral regurgitation (Chronic)	high pitched apical holosystolic radiates to axilla, S3 followed by short diastolic rumble	1st exertional dyspnea, atrial fib., emboli (20%), late parasternal lift (heave). ECG usually shows left atrial and ventricular hypertrophy.
Mitral stenosis	mid-diastolic apical, crescendos into S2, loud opening snap, loud S1	exertional dyspnea, orthopnea, hemoptysis, PACs, atrial fibrillation (40%), emboli (14%) , normal to low BP
Tricuspid regurgitation	high-pitched, pansystolic, at 4th para-sternal space	orthopnea, right sided failure (JVD, edema, large liver/spleen, ascites), ECG shows RBBB, or atrial fib.

Electrolyte Disorders

Criteria for Detecting Significant Electrolyte Abnormalities in ED Patients

Poor oral intake, vomiting	Recent seizures	Altered mental status
Hypertension, diuretic use	Muscle weakness	Recent abnormal
Age ≥ 65 years	Alcohol abuse	electrolytes

≥1 criteria had 95% sensitivity, 97% negative predictive value. *Ann Emerg Med* 1991;20:16.

CALCIUM

Hypocalcemia - Total calcium < 8.5 mg/dl or ionized Ca^{+2} < 2.0 mEq/L (1.0 mmol/L)
Hypercalcemia - Total calcium > 10.5 mg/dl or ionized Ca^{+2} > 2.7 mEq/L (1.3 mmol/L)
Hypoalbuminemia – a serum albumin ↓of 1 g/dl will↓ total serum Ca^{+2} 0.8 mg/dl

Hypocalcemia – Clinical Features

Symptoms	Physical Findings	Electrocardiogram
Paresthesias, fatigue	Hyperactive reflexes	• Prolonged QT
Seizures, tetany	Chvostek(C)/Trousseau(T) signs[1]	(esp. Ca^{+2} < 6.0 mg/dl)
Vomiting, weakness	Low blood pressure	• Bradycardia
Laryngospasm	Congestive heart failure	• Arrhythmias

[1]C–muscle twitch if tap facial nerve, T–carpal spasm after forearm BP cuff X 3 min

Hypocalcemia Evaluation

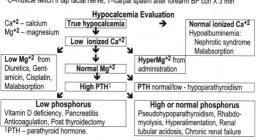

Ca^{+2} – calcium
Mg^{+2} – magnesium

True hypocalcemia → Normal ionized Ca^{+2}
Hypoalbuminemia:
  Nephrotic syndrome
  Malabsorption

Low ionized Ca^{+2}

Low Mg^{+2} from Diuretics, Gentamicin, Cisplatin, Malabsorption

Normal Mg^{+2}

HyperMg^{+2} from administration

High PTH[1]

PTH normal/low - hypoparathyroidism

Low phosphorus
Vitamin D deficiency, Pancreatitis Anticoagulation, Post thyroidectomy

High or normal phosphorus
Pseudohypoparathyroidism, Rhabdomyolysis, Hyperalimentation, Renal tubular acidosis, Chronic renal failure

[1]PTH – parathyroid hormone.

Drugs That Can Cause Hypocalcemia

• Cimetidine, Cisplatin	• Glucagon, Glucocorticoids	• Phosphates, Protamine
• Citrate (transfusion)	• Heparin	• Norepinephrine
• Dilantin, phenobarbital	• Loop diuretics (*Lasix*)	• Sodium nitroprusside
• Gentamicin, Tobramycin	• Magnesium sulfate	• Theophylline

Hypocalcemia Treatment

Drug	Preparation (elemental Ca+)	Drug Dose[1]
Ca gluconate	10% solution – 93 mg/ 10 ml	15-30 ml IV over 3-5 minutes
Ca chloride	10% solution – 273 mg/ 10ml	5 ml in 50 ml D5W IV over 10 min

[1] IV calcium may cause ↓BP, tissue necrosis, ↓HR or digoxin toxicity.
   Consider administration via central line, if possible to prevent extravasation risk.

<u>Hypercalcemia etiology</u>: (**PAM P SCHMIDT**) Hyper**P**arathyroidism, **A**ddison's disease, **M**ilk alkali syndrome, **P**aget's disease, **S**arcoid, **C**ancer, **H**yperthyroidism, **M**yeloma, **I**mmobilization, Hypervitaminosis **D**, **T**hiazides

Hypercalcemia – Clinical Features	
General	• Weakness, polydipsia, dehydration
Neurologic	• Confusion, irritability, hyporeflexia, headache
Skeletal	• Bone pain, fractures
Cardiac	• Hypertension, QT shortening, wide T wave, arrhythmias
GI	• Anorexia, weight loss, constipation, ulcer, pancreatitis
Renal	• Polyuria, renal insufficiency, nephrolithiasis

Hypercalcemia Evaluation

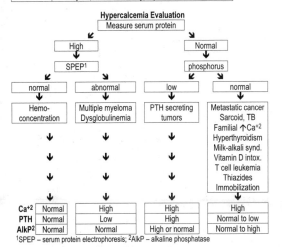

Ca^{+2}	Normal	High	High	High
PTH	Normal	Low	High	Normal to low
AlkP[2]	Normal	Normal	High or normal	Normal to high

[1]SPEP – serum protein electrophoresis; [2]AlkP – alkaline phosphatase

Hypercalcemia Management
- IV normal saline 1-2 Liters bolus, then 200-500 ml/hour
- Furosemide (*Lasix*) 10-40 mg IV q 2-4 h to keep urine output 200-300 ml/h
- Consider central line, and watch closely for signs of heart failure or overload
- Follow urine magnesium (Mg), and potassium (K^+) losses, replacing prn or empirically administering 15 mg Mg/hour and ≤ 10 mEq K^+/hour
- Consider dialysis with calcium free dialysate if renal failure
- EDTA at 10-50 mg/kg IV over 4 hours ONLY if life threatening features
- Other adjuncts: calcitonin, mithramycin, gallium, steroids

MAGNESIUM

Hypomagnesemia (<1.5 mEq/L): Due to alcohol, diuretics, aminoglycosides, malnourished. Irritable muscle, tetany, seizures. <u>Treat</u>: $MgSO_4$ 5-10 mg/kg IV over 20 min.

Hypermagnesemia (>2.2 mEq/L) Due to renal failure, excess maternal Mg supplement, or overuse of Mg-containing medicine. Clinical features: weakness, hyporeflexia, paralysis, and ECG with AV block and QT prolongation. <u>Treat</u>: Ca gluconate (10%) 10-20 ml IV.

POTASSIUM

Acute decreases in pH will increase K^+ (a $\downarrow$pH of 0.1 will $\uparrow K^+$ 0.3-1.3 mEq/L).

Causes of Hypokalemia	
• *Decreased K^+ intake* • *Intracellular shift* (normal stores): alkalemia, insulin, pseudohypokalemia of leukemia, familial hypokalemic periodic paralysis (HPP).	• *Increased excretion*: diuretics, hyperaldosteronism, penicillins (exchange Na^+/K^+), sweating, diarrhea (colonic fluid has high K^+), vomiting, binding in gut (clay ingestion – e.g. pica)

Hypokalemia Evaluation

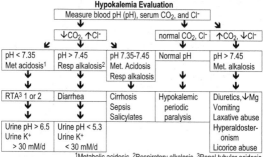

Measure blood pH (pH), serum CO_2, and Cl^-

$\downarrow CO_2$, $\uparrow Cl^-$		normal CO_2, Cl^-	$\uparrow CO_2$, $\downarrow Cl^-$
pH < 7.35 Met acidosis[1]	pH > 7.45 Resp alkalosis[2]	pH 7.35-7.45 Met. Acidosis Resp alkalosis	Normal pH	pH > 7.45 Met. alkalosis
RTA[3] 1 or 2	Diarrhea	Cirrhosis Sepsis Salicylates	Hypokalemic periodic paralysis	Diuretics, $\downarrow$Mg Vomiting Laxative abuse Hyperaldosteronism Licorice abuse
Urine pH > 6.5 Urine K^+ > 30 mM/d	Urine pH < 5.3 Urine K^+ < 30 mM/d			

[1]Metabolic acidosis, [2]Respiratory alkalosis, [3]Renal tubular acidosis

Clinical Features of Hypokalemia	Treatment of Hypokalemia
• Lethargy, confusion weakness • Areflexia, difficult respirations • Autonomic instability, Low BP	• Ensure adequate urine output first • Mild hypokalemia, replace orally only • Severe $\downarrow K^+$, use parenteral K^+ (e.g. cardiac, or neuromuscular symptoms or DKA).
ECG findings in Hypokalemia	
• $K^+ \leq 3.0$ mEq/L: low voltage QRS, flat T's, $\downarrow$ST, prominent P & U waves • $K^+ \leq 2.5$ mEq/L: prominent U waves • $K^+ \leq 2.0$ mEq/L: widened QRS	• Administer K^+ at ≤ 10 mEq/h using ≤ 40 mEq/L while on cardiac monitor. • 40 mEq raises serum K^+ by 1 mEq/L

Hyperkalemia

Causes of Hyperkalemia

- *Pseudohyperkalemia* due to blood sampling or hemolysis.
- *Exogenous*: blood, salt substitutes, potassium containing drugs (e.g. penicillin derivatives), acute digoxin toxicity, β blockers, succinylcholine.

- *Endogenous* – acidemia, trauma, burns, rhabdomyolysis, DIC, sickle cell crisis, GI bleed, chemotherapy (destroying tumor mass), mineralo-corticoid deficiency), congenital defects (21 hydroxylase deficiency)

Hyperkalemia Evaluation

Measure CO_2 and Cl^-

↙ ↘

| Low serum CO_2 | Normal CO_2 and Cl^- |

↓ ↓

| Serum pH < 7.35 Metabolic acidosis | Serum pH 7.35-7.45 |

↓ ↓

- Renal failure
- Hypoaldosteronism (e.g. Addison's)
- Diabetic Ketoacidosis

- Insulin deficiency & hyperglycemia
- Pseudohyperkalemia (e.g. high WBC or high platelets)

Clinical Features of Hyperkalemia	Treatment of Hyperkalemia
• Paresthesias, weakness • Ascending paralysis sparing head, trunk, and respiration.	• Calcium gluconate[1] (10%)–5-30 ml IV over 2-5 min, may repeat **OR** • CaCl$_2$[1] (10%) 5-10 ml IV over 5-10 min • NaHCO$_3$[2] 1 mEq/kg IV, repeat ½ dose q 10 min prn • Glucose/Insulin – 10 units regular insulin IV + 1 amp D$_{50}$ IV, then 10-20 units regular insulin in 500 ml D10W IV over 1 h if needed • Albuterol nebulizer 10-20 mg over 15 min, may repeat • Furosemide 40-80 mg IV • Kayexalate[2] 15-60 g PO or 50 g PR • Dialysis

ECG in Hyperkalemia (K^+ in mEq/L)	
K^+	ECG findings
> 5.5-6	Peaked T waves
> 6-6.5	↑ PR and QT intervals
> 6.5-7	flat or isoelectric P waves, ↓ ST segments
> 7-7.5	↑intraventricular conduction
> 7.5-8	↑ QRS, ST&T waves merge
> 10.0	sine wave appearance

[1] Contraindicated if digoxin toxicity. IV CaCl$_2$ can cause phlebitis.
[2] May worsen fluid overload (i.e. congestive heart failure)

SODIUM

FE_{Na} = fraction of Na^+ in urine filtered by the glomerulus and not reabsorbed.

FE_{Na} = 100 x (urine Na^+/plasma Na^+) ÷ (urine creatinine/plasma creatinine)

Hyponatremia

Na^+ = falsely ↓ 1.6 mEq/L for each 100 mg/dL ↑ in glucose over 100 mg/dL.

Clinical Features of Hyponatremia	
• Lethargy, apathy, Cerebral edema	• Seizures, Hypothermia
• Depressed reflexes, muscle cramps	• Pseudobulbar palsies

Hyponatremia Evaluation

Deficit body Na^+ > deficit body water		Excess total body water (no edema)	Excess total body water > excess Na^+ (edema)	
Renal losses: diuretics, mineralocorticoid deficiency, salt losing nephritis, bicarbonaturia, ketonuria, osmotic diuresis	*Extrarenal loss*: vomit, diarrhea, 3rd space fluids, pancreatitis, peritonitis, traumatized muscle	Glucocorticoid deficiency, low thyroid, pain, emotional stress, drugs, (SIADH - U_{osm} usually > S_{osm})	Nephrotic syndrome, cirrhosis, CHF	Acute and chronic renal failure

(Obtain urine Na^+, urine creatinine, urine osmolality, and serum osmolality)

Na^+>20 mEq/L ↑FE_{Na}, ↓ SG[1] U_{osm}[3] varies	Na^+<10 mEq/L ↓FE_{Na}, ↑ SG[1] U_{osm}[3] > 800	Na^+>20 mEq/L Nl[2] FE_{Na}, ↑ SG[1] U_{osm}[3] varies	Na^+<10 mEq/L ↓FE_{Na}, ↑ SG[1] high U_{osm}[3]	Na^+>20 mEq/L ↑FE_{Na}, ↓ SG[1] U_{osm}[3] varies
		Management		
Isotonic saline	Isotonic saline	Water restrict	Water restrict	Water restrict

[1] SG – specific gravity, [2] Nl– normal, [3] U_{osm} – urine osmolality, [4] S_{osm} -serum osmolality

Hypertonic Saline Administration (3% NaCl = 513 mEq/L)

Indication	• Severe ↓ Na^+ with serious CNS manifestations (e.g. seizures)
Goal	• Only ↑Na^+ to 120-125 mEq/L acutely,& maximum of 12 mEq/L/24h.
Formula	• Na^+ deficit = weight (kg) X 0.6 X (desired Na^+[~125] – known Na^+) • Infusion rate (ml/hour) that will ↑Na^+ 1 mEq/L/hour = (weight [kg] X 0.6) ÷ (0.513 mEq/L X 1 hour)
Rate	• 2-4 mEq/L/hour - if active seizing, or ↑ intracranial pressure over 1 hour or until seizing stops, then ↓ rate to 1-2 mEq/L/hour • 1-2 mEq/L/hour - if obtunded, or other neurologic symptoms
Adjuncts	• Furosemide (*Lasix*) – 40 mg IV; remember to check Na^+ q 2 hours

Hypernatremia

Clinical Features of Hypernatremia	
• Lethargy, irritability, coma	• Doughy skin
• Seizures	• Late preservation of intravascular
• Spasticity, hyperreflexia	volume (and vital signs)

Hypernatremia Etiology, Diagnosis and Management

$Na^+ + H_2O$ loss with low total body Na^+		H_2O loss with normal total body Na^+		Excess Na^+ with increased total body Na^+
Renal losses osmotic diuresis (mannitol, glucose, urea)	Extrarenal loss excess sweat, diarrhea	Renal loss diabetes insipidus (nephrogenic, central) Serum osm > 295 mosm/L, Serum Na^+ > 145 mEq/L, U_{osm} < 150 mosm/L	Extrarenal loss Respiratory and skin loss	Primary hyper-aldosteronism, Cushing's syndrome, hypertonic dialysis, hypertonic Na^+ bicarbonate, NaCl tablets

Diagnosis				
BUN normal,↑ U Na^+>20 mEq/L, U_{osm} hypotonic	BUN ↑ U Na^+<10 mEq/L, U_{osm} > 600-800 mosm/L	BUN ± normal U Na^+ varies U_{osm} often < 100-150 mosm/L in central DI	BUN ↑ U Na^+ varies U_{osm} > 600-800 mOsm/L	BUN ± normal U Na^+>20 mEq/L U_{osm} isotonic or hypertonic

Management				
Hypotonic saline	Hypotonic saline	Water replacement D_5W	Water replacement D_5W	Diuretic+H_2O replacement D_5W

[1] U-urine, U_{osm} – urine osmolality

Management of Hypernatremia

- Correct hypernatremia slowly over 48 to 72 hours. Overvigorous rehydration can cause cerebral edema, seizures, coma, or death. Lower Na^+ no faster than 1-2 mEq/L/hour.
- With endogenous Na^+ overload, treatment consists of salt restriction and correction of the primary underlying disorder. If there is excess exogenous mineralocorticoid, restrict salt and modify replacement therapy.

Endocrine Disorders

Adrenal Insufficiency

Clinical Features		Adrenal Crisis Therapy
Weakness	99%	• 1-2 Liters NS IV with further IV fluids as needed
↑pigment	92%	• Correct electrolyte abnormalities
Weight loss	97%	• Hydrocortisone (*Solu-Cortef*) 200 mg IV, + 100 mg q8h
Vomiting	70%	or dexamethasone 4 mg IV (will not interfere with ACTH
Anorexia	98%	stimulation testing)
BP < 110/70	85%	• If possible draw & store blood for steroid level analysis
Abdominal		including baseline serum cortisol and ACTH levels.
Pain	34%	• Consider broad spectrum antibiotics (e.g. ceftriaxone 1-
Salt craving	22%	2 g IV) if suspicion of sepsis
Diarrhea	20%	• Perform rapid bedside check of blood sugar
↑ K+		• Treat underling precipitants (e.g. sepsis, hypothermia,
↓ Na+		MI,↓glucose, bleeding, trauma, remove meds that
Eosinophilia		↓cortisone: morphine, chlorpromazine, barbiturates)

Diabetes Mellitus

Sliding Scale Insulin Regimen for Type II Diabetes
- If taking PO, monitor blood glucose 30 minutes before meals and qhs. If taking PO continue normal maintenance insulin in addition to sliding scale detailed below. Typical maintenance (0.5-1.0 Unit/kg/day divided 2/3 in AM and 1/3 in PM)
- If not taking PO, monitor blood glucose q 6 hours (6AM,12PM, 6 PM, 12AM) and use sliding scale detailed below.

Glucose (mg/dl)	Low dose Insulin (elderly or underweight)	Medium dose Insulin (average weight patients)	High dose Insulin (overweight patients)	Very High dose (steroids or infection)
< 60	Treat hypoglycemia			
60-150	0	0	0	0
151-200	2 units	4 units	6 units	8 units
201-250	4 units	6 units	8 units	10 units
251-300	6 units	8 units	10 units	12 units
301-350	8 units	10 units	12 units	14 units
351-400	10 units	12 units	14 units	16 units
> 400	12 units[1]	14 units[1]	16 units[1]	18 units[1]

Advance to next higher insulin dose if glucose > 250 mg/dl in 24 hours AND all levels > 100 mg/dl. Decrease to next lower insulin dose if blood glucose 60-100 mg/dl at least twice in a 24 hour period.
[1]Evaluate for precipitant/complication (infection, acidosis, stroke, other disease)

INSULIN	Preparation	Onset (h)	Peak (h)	Duration (h)
Rapid acting	Regular	0.5-1	2.5-5	8-12
	Lispro (*Humalog*)	0.25	0.5-1.5	2-5
	Aspart (*Novolog*)	0.25	1-3	3-5
Intermediate acting	NPH	1-1.5	4-12	24
	Lente	1-2.5	7-15	24
Long acting	Glargine (*Lantus*)	slow prolonged absorption[1]		
	Ultralente	4-8	10-30	20-36

Humulin + *Novolin* 70/30, 50/50 preparations = %NPH/%regular insulin.
[1]Relatively constant concentration/time profile over 24 h with no pronounced peak.

Diabetic Ketoacidosis (DKA)

Laboratory diagnosis of DKA	Precipitants of DKA	
• Blood glucose > 300 mg/dl	• Recent change in insulin dose	40%
• Serum bicarbonate < 15 mEq/L in the absence of chronic renal failure	• Infection	40%
	• Noncompliance (diet or meds)	23%
• Serum acetone level > 2:1 dilution	• Trauma, injury, and stroke	10%
• Arterial pH < 7.30 in 1st 24 hours	• No prior diabetes	20%

[1] DKA occasionally occurs with blood glucose below 300 mg/dl – especially in patients
taking exogenous insulin. *Am J Epidemiol* 1983; 117: 551.

DKA Management

- Apply cardiac monitor and administer O_2 if altered mental status or shock.
- Obtain labs and assess for DKA precipitants or complications.
- <u>IV fluids</u> – IV NS until hypotension, and orthostasis resolve. (a) if corrected serum Na is normal or high, administer ½NS at 4-14 ml/kg/hour depending on hydration status. (b) if corrected Na is low, administer NS at 4-14 ml/kg/hour depending on hydration status.
- <u>Insulin</u> – 0.15 U/kg (U) regular insulin IV, then 0.1 U/kg/h IV. If serum glucose, does not fall by 50-70 mg/dl in first hour double insulin infusion hourly until glucose falls 50-70 mg/dl in hour. When glucose falls to 250 mg/dl, change IV to D5 ½NS at 150-250 ml/hour with adequate insulin (0.05 – 0.1 U/kg/hour) to keep glucose between 150-200 mg/dl until metabolic control achieved. Change to SC regular insulin once bicarbonate is > 15 mEq/L and no anion gap.
- <u>Replace potassium</u> (1st verify adequate urine output).
  (a) If initial K^+ is normal or low, add 10-40 mEq K^+/L to IV fluids. Some authorities recommend replacing K^+ with 2:1 mix of KCL and K_3PO_4. Some authorities recommend holding insulin until K^+ rises to > 3.3 mEq/L. (b) If initial K^+ is high, hold K^+, check levels q 2h, then add K, when it falls to normal.
- <u>Bicarbonate</u> – primarily indicated for hyperkalemia management, if needed.
  Diabetes Care 2004, 27 Suppl 1:S94-102.

Hyperosmolar Hyperglycemic Nonketotic Coma (HHNC)

Diagnosis of HHNC	Etiology/Precipitants of HHNC	
• Plasma osmolarity > 350 mOsm/L	Renal failure	Pancreatitis
• Glucose > 600 mg/dl	Pneumonia, Sepsis	Burn
• No ketosis (lactic acidosis ± present)	GI bleed	Heat stroke
• 50-65% have no history of diabetes	MI	Dialysis
• ↑ BUN with BUN/Cr ratio > 30	CNS bleed/stroke	Recent surgery
• ↑ CK due to rhabdomyolysis	Pulmonary emboli	Medicines[1]

[1]Thiazides, Ca^{+2} channel blocker, steroids, phenytoin, propranolol, furosemide, cimetidine, chlorthalidone, loxapine.

History		Physical Exam	
Fever	Polydipsia	↓consciousness	Hemiparesis
Thirst	Confusion	Tachycardia, ↓BP	Myoclonus
Polyuria or	Seizures (focal)	Fever	Quadriplegia
Oliguria	Hallucinations	Focal seizure	Nystagmus

Management
• Admit all patients to the ICU, and consider placement of central line.
• Obtain electrolytes, CK, UA, CXR, ECG, cultures, ± head CT and spinal tap.
• <u>Fluids</u>- mean fluid deficit is 9 L. Start IV NS until BP & urine output OK. Then, change to ½NS & replace 50% of deficit over 12 h, & 50% over next 12-24 h.
• <u>Add dextrose</u> (D5½NS) once glucose falls ≤ 300 mg/dl.
• <u>Replace potassium</u> (5-10 mEq per h) when level available & OK urine output.
• <u>Insulin</u> may be unnecessary. Consider single 0.1 U/kg IV dose with 0.05 U/kg/hr IV until glucose is 300 mg/dl.
Empiric phosphate repletion, subcutaneous heparin and broad-spectrum prophylactic antibiotics may be needed depending upon clinical circumstances.

Hypoglycemia

Etiology	Clinical Features
Fasting hypoglycemia Symptoms begin 4-6 h after meal. (1) overuse (drugs, insulin, sepsis, tumors, starvation, exercise) or (2) underproduction (alcohol, β blockers, salicylate, hormone deficiency, liver or renal failure, enzyme defects, or substrate defects as in malnutrition). *Reactive hypoglycemia* within 1-2 h of meal & due to impaired GI motility, impaired glucose tolerance (?early diabetes), or enzyme defect.	*Sympathetic response*: ↑HR, hunger, tremors, or sweating. These may be absent if diabetes, alcohol abuse, or β blocker use. *Neuronal dysfunction*: headache, coma, seizures, focal deficits.

Management
• Glucose 1 amp (50 ml) of $D_{50}W$ IV (↑glucose ~ 150 mg/dl) or glucagon 1 mg IM/SC if no IV. IV D_5NS or $D_{10}NS$ to maintain normal blood glucose if needed.
• Diazoxide (*Hyperstat*) 1-2 mg/kg IV if unable to control with IV glucose.
• Octreotide – may be more useful than Diazoxide for sulfonylurea hypoglycemia. Administer via IV infusion or SC dosing. Contact poison center for dosing.
• Hydrocortisone (*Solu-Cortef*) 100 mg IV if possible adrenal insufficiency.
• Thiamine 100 mg IV or IM if malnourished.
• Admit all intentional oral hypoglycemic and insulin overdoses.
• If mild unintentional insulin overdose, administer D50 or oral glucose, feed meal, observe for a short time period and discharge.
• If mild unintentional short acting oral agent overdose, no recurrent symptoms over 6-8 h, and charcoal given, some recommend discharge. Otherwise admit all oral hypoglycemic overdoses due to prolonged hypoglycemic effects.

Hyperthyroidism/Thyroid Storm

Underlying Thyroid Disease	Precipitants of Thyroid Storm	
• Grave's disease (most common)	Infection (#1)	Iodine therapy/dye
• Toxic nodular goiter	Pulmonary embolus	Stroke
• Toxic adenoma	DKA, or HHNC	Surgery
• Factitious thyrotoxicosis	Thyroid hormone	Childbirth
• Excess TSH	excess	D&C

Clinical Features of Thyroid Storm (Thyrotoxicosis)		
Hyperkinesis	Temperature > 101 F	Psychosis, apathy, coma
Palpable goiter	↑HR + ↑pulse pressure	Tremor, hyperreflexia
Proptosis, lid lag	Arrhythmia (new onset)[2]	Diarrhea, weight loss
Exophthalmos, palsy[1]	Palpitations, dyspnea	Jaundice

[1]Palsy of extraocular muscles, [2]Atrial fibrillation/flutter which may be refractory to digoxin

Laboratory Features of Thyrotoxicosis[1]	• $\uparrow$freeT$_4$, $\uparrow$T$_3$, $\downarrow$TSH • $\uparrow$T$_4$RIA, $\uparrow$FT$_4$I	• $\uparrow$glucose,$\uparrow$Ca^{+2},$\downarrow$Hb, $\uparrow$WBC,$\downarrow$cholesterol

[1]Laboratory tests can diagnose hyperthyroidism, but thyrotoxicosis is a clinical diagnosis.

Treatment

- Supportive care, O$_2$,✓ glucose, fever control (avoid aspirin) & treat precipitants.
- <u>Inhibit thyroid hormone synthesis:</u> *Propylthiouracil* (PTU) 600-900 mg PO on day 1, then 300-400 mg/d PO X 3-6 weeks. PTU inhibits conversion of T$_4$ to T$_3$.
- <u>Inhibit thyroid hormone release:</u> K$^+$ iodide as *Lugol's solution* (8 mg iodide/drop) - 1 ml or 20 drops PO q 8 h. **OR** *SSKI* (40 mg iodide/drop) 2-10 drops PO daily. **OR** *Na$^+$ iodide* 1 g IV q 8-12 hours (give over 30 min). **Caution:** Administer iodide $\geq$ 1 h after anti-thyroid medications to prevent use in hormone synthesis.
- <u>Blockade of peripheral effects:</u> Propranolol 1 mg slowly IV q 15 min (Max 5 mg) prn to reduce sympathetic hyperactivity and conversion of T$_4$ to T$_3$. Begin propranolol 20-120 mg PO q 6-8 hours when symptoms improve.
- <u>Inhibit conversion of T4 to T3:</u> hydrocortisone (*Solu-Cortef*) 100 mg IV q 8h.

Apathetic Thyrotoxicosis

A rare form of thyrotoxicosis usually occurring in the elderly.

Clinical Features		Management
• Mean age > 60 years • Lethargy, $\downarrow$ mentation • No Grave's eye signs • Smaller goiter • Depression/apathy	• Weak proximal muscles • Mean weight loss > 40 lb. • Atrial fibrillation (in 75%) • Congestive heart failure • Atrial fibrillation/CHF may be refractory to treatment	Treat as thyro-toxicosis but use lower doses and slower rates as side effects are greater in elderly.

Hypothyroidism/Myxedema Coma

Precipitants of Myxedema Coma		Lab tests
Pneumonia, GI bleed CHF, cold exposure Stroke, trauma, $\downarrow$glucose $\downarrow$pO$_2$,$\uparrow$pCO$_2$, $\downarrow$Na$^+$	*Drugs* Phenothiazines, lithium, narcotics, sedatives, phenytoin, propranolol	Serum TSH > 60 µU/ml $\downarrow$ total & free T4 $\downarrow$ or $\leftrightarrow$ total & free T3

Clinical Features of Myxedema Coma	
Vitals	• Temperature is often < 90 F, 50% have BP < 100/60
Cardiac	• $\downarrow$HR, heart block, low voltage, ST-T changes, $\uparrow$Q-T, effusion
Pulmonary	• Hypoventilation, $\uparrow$pCO$_2$, $\downarrow$O$_2$, pleural effusions
Metabolic	• Hyponatremia, hypoglycemia
Neurologic	• Coma, seizures, tremors, ataxia, nystagmus, psychiatric disturbances. Depressed or "hung up" reflexes
GI/GU	• Ileus, ascites, fecal impaction, megacolon, urinary retention
Skin	• Alopecia, loss of lateral 1/3 eyebrows, nonpitting puffiness around eyes, hands, and pretibial region of legs
ENT	• Tongue enlarges, voice deepens and becomes hoarse

Management of Myxedema Coma

- Administer O_2, rewarm and treat cause (e.g. infection, $\downarrow$ glucose).
- Thyroxine – 400-500 µg slow IV on day 1, + 50-100 µg IV q day. **CAUTION** IV thyroxine may cause cardiac arrest. Reduce dose if cardiac ischemia or arrhythmias. Some experts recommend no IV thyroxine for 3-7 days after day 1.
- Start oral thyroxine 100-200 µg PO q day when possible.
- Hydrocortisone (*Solu-Cortef*) 100 mg IV q 8h.

Environmental Disorders

Scuba Diving Injuries (Dysbarism)

Dysbaric air embolism (DAE): gas bubbles enter circulation through ruptured pulmonary veins causing symptoms within 10 minutes of surfacing. Symptoms: cardiac arrest, seizure, cardiac ischemia, stroke, and asymmetric multiplegias.
Decompression sickness (DCS): formation of gas bubbles in blood and body tissues following $\downarrow$ in ambient pressure. $\uparrow$ risk with old age, obesity, dehydration, alcohol use, exercise, unpressurized flight after dive. Symptoms occur 10 min-6 h (rarely delayed 24-48 h) after ascent and are due to bubbles causing vascular occlusion.
<u>Type I DCS</u> involves lymphatics, skin (mottled rash, itching), musculoskeletal (periarticular joint pain worse with movement) esp. shoulders and elbows.
<u>Type II DCS</u> causes neurologic disruption with spinal cord involvement (low thoracic, lumbar, and sacral primarily) with paraplegia, and bladder dysfunction. Pulmonary involvement with pain, dyspnea, and edema may occur.

DCS and DAE Management

- 100% O_2 & IV NS unless contraindicated. Exclude injuries (e.g. pneumothorax).
- Do not place in Trendelenberg. This worsens CNS edema and dyspnea.
- Transport to nearest hyperbaric recompression chamber. If uncertain where nearest facility is call **(919) 684-8111**. Must fly at low altitude < 1000 feet or use aircraft that can pressurize to 1 atmosphere (ATA).

High Altitude Syndromes

Acute Mountain Sickness – AMS

Risk factors: rapid ascent, high sleeping altitudes, 25% > 6900 feet (2000 meters), low vital capacity, low hypoxic ventilatory response (COPD).
Clinical Features: Early: lightheadedness, breathlessness, hangover (headache, anorexia, vomiting, irritable, sleepy), & later dyspnea, oliguria, high altitude cerebral/pulmonary edema (20% local rales), retinal hemorrhages > 5000 meters
Prevention: acetazolamide or dexamethasone 24 h preascent + 2 d after ascent.

Acute Mountain Sickness Management	
Acute Mountain Sickness Management	• Stop ascent or descend if worsening, O_2 0.5-1 L/min at night
	• Acetazolamide (*Diamox*) 125-250 mg PO bid
	• Dexamethasone (*Decadron*) 4 mg PO q6h
	• Hyperbaric oxygen therapy (e.g. hyperbaric bag)

High Altitude Syndromes

High Altitude Cerebral Edema - HACE

Progressive neurologic deterioration in someone with HAPE or AMS.
Clinical Features: altered mental status, ataxia, stupor and coma if untreated.
Headache and vomiting are not always present. Focal deficits may occur.

High Altitude Cerebral Edema Management	• Immediate descent or evacuation, supplemental O_2
	• Dexamethasone (*Decadron*) 8 mg PO, IM, or IV then 4 mg q 6h
	• Acetazolamide (*Diamox*) 125 mg PO bid
	• If coma, intubation. Hyperventilation only if acute deterioration
	• Furosemide (*Lasix*) 40-80 mg IV (avoid dehydration, & ↓BP)
	• Hyperbaric oxygen therapy (e.g. hyperbaric bag)

High Altitude Pulmonary Edema - HAPE

Risk factors: male sex, child, exertion, rapid ascent, cold, excess salt, sleeping medications, prior HAPE/AMS. HAPE is a noncardiogenic edema due to exaggerated pulmonary pressor response to hypoxia.
Clinical Features: dry cough, poor exercise, local rales, and later development of tachycardia, tachypnea, dyspnea, cyanosis, generalized rales, and coma. AMS need not be present. A right ventricular heave may be noted. ECG ± right axis deviation, RV strain. CXR may show cephalization or pulmonary edema.

High Altitude Pulmonary Edema Management	• Immediate descent (with minimal exertion), warming, O_2
	• Hyperbarics, morphine 2-5 mg, furosemide (*Lasix*) 40-80 mg IV
	• CPAP or BiPAP (see page 132)
	• Nifedipine (*Procardia*) 10 mg PO reduces pulmonary artery pressure by 30-50% & ↑O_2 saturation. Nifedipine (extended release) 30 mg PO q8h may prophylax against HAPE.

Hyperthermia and Hypothermia

Minor Heat Illness

- *Heat Syncope*: Postural hypotension from vasodilation, volume depletion, and ↓ vascular tone. Rehydrate, remove from heat, and evaluate for serious disease.
- *Heat cramps*: Painful, contractions of calves, thigh, or shoulders in those who are sweating liberally and drinking hypotonic solutions (e.g. water). Replace fluids: 0.1-0.2% oral solution or IV NS rehydration. Do not use salt tablets.
- *Heat Exhaustion*: Salt and water depletion causing orthostasis, and hyperthermia (usually < 104F). Mental status, and neurologic exam are normal. Lab: high hematocrit, high sodium, or high BUN. Treat with NS 1-2 Liters IV.

Heatstroke

Clinical Features	Risk Factors

• Hyperpyrexia (>104-105.8F/40-41C)
• Central nervous system dysfunction (seizures, altered mentation, plantar responses, hemiplegia, ataxia)
• Loss of sweating (variably present)
• ↓ Na, ↓ Ca, ↓ phosphate, ↓ or ↑ K
• Rhabdomyolysis, renal/liver failure
	• Old age, skin disorders, obesity
	• Drugs
	  - amphetamines
	  - anticholinergics
	  - antihypertensive agents
	  - sympathomimetics (e.g. cocaine)
	  - phenothiazines

Management of Heatstroke

- Administer oxygen, protect airway if comatose or seizing. Check blood glucose.
- Measure temperature with continuous rectal probe accurate at high levels.
- Begin IV NS cautiously as pulmonary edema is common and mean fluid requirement is only 1.2 L in first 4 hours. Consider central line pressures as guide.
- Immediate cooling by: (1) *evaporation*: Spray with tepid water and direct fan at patient (0.1 - 0.3C/min temp. drop). For shivering, IV lorazepam 1-3 mg IV. (2) *ice water (or 60F) tub immersion*: (controversial) (temp. drop ~ 0.16C/min). (3) *Ice packs, cooling blankets, peritoneal dialysis, gastric lavage* with cold saline are slow or unproven. (4) Avoid aspirin (hyperpyrexia). Avoid repeated Tylenol doses (possible liver damage and ineffective in heatstroke).
- Stop above measures at temperature of 102-104°F to avoid over-correction.
- Place Foley catheter to monitor urine output (see rhabdomyolysis below).
- Obtain CBC, electrolytes, renal function, glucose, liver enzymes, LDH/CK, PT, and PTT, arterial blood gas, and fibrin degradation products. ECG and CXR.
- Exclude other fever cause: infection, malignant hyperthermia, thyroid, drugs etc.

Other Heat Related Disorders

- **Malignant hyperthermia (MH):** Autosomal dominant disorder causing fever, & rigid muscles after anesthetics or succinylcholine is administered.
  <u>*Treatment*</u>: Stop agent, lower temp. as in heatstroke (avoid phenothiazines), give dantrolene 2-3 mg/kg IV q 6 hours (max cumulative dose is 10 mg/kg).

- **Neuroleptic Malignant Syndrome:** Similar to MH with fever, muscle rigidity, and altered mentation, but due to anticholinergics (e.g. phenothiazines).
  <u>*Treatment:*</u> Stop agent, treat heat stroke (avoid phenothiazines) and administer benzodiazepines IV (e.g. lorazepam). Many authorities recommend (1) dantrolene 2-3 mg/kg IV then continuous infusion until symptoms subside or maximum dose of 10 mg/kg plus (2) bromocriptine 2.5-10 mg PO tid. (However, use of dantrolene and bromocriptine is controversial as one study [20 total patients] found their use prolonged illness and increased adverse sequelae, *Br J Psychiatry* 1991;159:709)

Other Heat Related Disorders Continued

- **Rhabdomyolysis:** Syndrome with release of contents into circulation due to tissue hypoxia, direct injury, exercise, enzyme defects, metabolic disease (DKA, ↓ K, ↓ Na, or ↓ phosphate, thyroid), toxins, infections, heatstroke.
  Complications[1]: renal failure, ↑K+, ↑Ca+2 or↓ Ca+2, ↑or↓phosphate, ↑ uric acid, compartment syndrome, disseminated intravascular coagulation.
  Treatment: (1) IV NS to keep urine output > 100-200 ml/hr, (2) NaHCO3 ≥ 50 mEq IV to keep urine pH > 6.5, (3) If poor urine output, administer Mannitol – 25-50 g IV,+ 12.5 g to each L of NS, (4) Dialyze if ↑K+ or uremia is present

- **Serotonin syndrome** – see page 164

[1] R = 0.7 [K+ in mEq/L] + 1.1 [Creatinine in mg/dl] + 0.6 [albumin in g/dl] – 6.6;
A single retrospective study found that a R ≥ 0.1 had a 41% risk of myoglobinuria induced renal failure, while a R < 0.1 had a 0% risk.   *Medicine* 1982; 3: 141.

HYPOTHERMIA

Severity	Temp. F (C)		Features
Mild	91-95 (33-35)		Maximal shivering + slurred speech at 95F
Moderate	85-90 (29-32)		At 89 – altered mental status, mydriasis, shivering ceases, muscles are rigid, incoordination, bradypnea
Severe	≤ 82	(≤ 28)	Bradycardia in 50%, Osborne waves on ECG, voluntary motion stops, pupils are fixed dilated
	79	(26)	Loss of consciousness, areflexia, no pain response
	77	(25)	No respirations, appear dead, pulmonary edema
	68	(20)	Asystole

Management of Hypothermia

- No vigorous manipulation or active external rewarming unless mild hypothermia.
- Evaluate for cause (e.g. sepsis, hypoglycemia, CNS disease, adrenal crisis).
- **Mild hypothermia** (> 32C): Administer humidified warmed O_2. Passive external rewarming and treatment of underlying disease is often only treatment needed.
- **Moderate hypothermia** (29-32C): Active internal rewarming. Drugs and cardioversion for cardiac arrest may be ineffective. Warm humidified O_2, with gastric or peritoneal lavage if < 1C/hour temp. rise. CPR, & advanced life support prn.
- **Severe hypothermia** (≤ 29 C): (1) Warm humidified O_2, warm IV fluids. (2) If nonarrested, warm peritoneal dialysis (41C dialysate), or (3) pleural irrigation (41C). (4) If core temperature < 25C consider femoral-femoral bypass. (5) Use open pleural lavage for direct cardiac rewarming if core temperature < 28C after 1 h of bypass in an arrest rhythm. If signs of life, and non-arrested, avoid CPR, and ACLS. If arrested, CPR and ACLS are OK. (6) Do not treat atrial arrhythmias. (7) Treat ↓BP with NS 1st. Use pressors cautiously. (8) Consider empiric D_{50}, thiamine 100 mg IV, *Narcan* 2mg IV, + hydrocortisone 100 mg IV.

Snake Bite Envenomation

(Crotalid) Snakebite Severity Score (for serial snake bite evaluation)

System	Manifestations	Points
Lung	No symptoms/signs	0
	Dyspnea, tight chest, mild discomfort, respiratory rate (RR) 20-25	1
	Moderate distress (RR 26-30, accessory muscle use)	2
	Cyanosis, air hunger, RR > 30, respiratory insufficiency/failure	3
Cardiac	No symptoms/signs	0
	Heart rate (HR) 100-125, palpitations, generally weak, ↑BP	1
	HR 126-175, systolic blood pressure (SBP) > 100 mm Hg	2
	HR > 175, SPB < 100, malignant dysrhythmia, cardiac arrest	3
Wound	No symptoms/signs	0
	Pain, swelling, ecchymosis within 5-7.5 cm of wound	1
	Pain, swelling, ecchymosis < ½ extremity (7.5-50 cm from bite)	2
	Pain, swelling, ecchymosis ½ to all extremity 50-100 cm from bite	3
	Pain, swelling, ecchymosis beyond extremity > 100 cm from bite	4
GI	No symptoms/signs	0
	Pain, tenesmus, or nausea	1
	Vomiting or diarrhea	2
	Repeated vomiting, diarrhea, hematemesis, hematochezia	3
Blood[2]	No symptoms/signs	0
	PT < 20, PTT < 50, Plat. (100-150k), Fbg. 100-150 µg/ml	1
	PT 20-50, PTT 50-75, Plat. (50-100k), Fbg. 50-100 µg/ml	2
	PT 50-100, PTT 75-100, Plat. (20-50k), Fbg. < 50 µg/ml	3
	PT/PTT/Fbg unmeasurable, Plat < 20k, serious bleeding risk	4
CNS	No symptoms/signs	0
	Mild apprehension, headache, weak, dizzy, chills, paresthesias	1
	Above plus confusion, or fasciculation in area of bite	2
	Severe confusion, seizure, coma, psychosis, gen. fasciculation	3

Ann Emerg Med 2001; 37: 175; & 1996; 27: 321.

Snakebite Grades (for dosing Polyvalent Equine Crotalid Antivenin)

Grade[1]	Features of Crotalid (Pit viper) envenomation	Dose
None 1.3 ± 0.5	± Fang marks, no pain, erythema or systemic symptoms	None
Mild[2] 2.1 ± 0.2	Fang marks, mild pain/edema, no systemic symptoms	0-5 vials (50 ml)
Moderate 3.2 ± 0.3	Fang marks, severe pain, moderate edema in 1st 12h, mild symptoms (vomiting, paresthesias), mild coagulopathy (without bleeding)	10 vials (100 ml)
Severe 8.5 ± 1.0	Fang marks, severe pain/edema, severe symptoms (hypotension, dyspnea), coagulopathy with bleeding	15-20 vials (150-200 ml)

[1] Correlation of Grade and Snakebite Severity Score

[2] Controversial – some experts recommend no antivenin for mild envenomation.

Prehospital Treatment for Crotalid Envenomation

- Decrease patient movement, and transport to nearest medical facility.
- Immobilize extremity in neutral position below level of heart.
- Incision + drainage and tourniquets are unproven and not recommended.

Emergency Treatment for Crotalid Envenomation

- Perform exam, measure envenomation site, and administer fluids, pressors prn.
- If no signs of envenomation, clean wound, administer tetanus and observe for a minimum of 6 hours. Consider antibiotics (e.g. *Augmentin* X 5 days).
- If significant envenomation, obtain CBC, electrolytes, renal and liver function tests, PT, PTT, fibrinogen, urinalysis, ECG, and type and cross.
- Choose Equine or Ovine Antivenin based on availability. Ovine is preferred.

Ovine - Crotalidae Polyvalent Immune Fab Antivenin (FabAV)

- Sheep derived antivenin that is 5X more potent than equine antivenin with less risk of allergy/anaphylaxis.
- Regardless of grade administer initial dose of 6 vials.
- Administer an additional 2 vials at 6, 12, and 18 hours.
- Dilute FabAV to a total of 250 ml in NS & infuse IV over one hour.
- Review package insert for further recommendations *Ann Emerg Med* 2001; 37:181.

Equine - Antivenin Crotalidae Polyvalent Administration - see dose prior page

- Perform skin test only if equine to be administered: 0.2 ml SC (dilute 1:10 with NS) at site distant from bite. Observe for allergy ≥ 10 minutes after injection. Absence of reaction does not exclude allergy.
- Need for antivenin and specific dose is controversial. Prior to administration, obtain consent, administer IV NS, consider premedication with diphenhydramine 1 mg/kg IV, and dilute antivenin in 50-100 ml each vial.
- Reconstitute antivenin in a 1:10 solution with NS or D_5W.
- Administer 5-10 ml over 5 min. If no allergy, increase rate so that infusion takes 1-2 hours. If symptoms progress, additional antivenin may be required.
- If allergic reaction and antivenin is necessary, start arterial line, continue to treat with NS ± albumin, methylprednisolone 125 mg IV, and diphenhydramine 50 mg IV. Hang epinephrine drip in line separate from antivenin (e.g. 0.6mg/kg epi 1:1,000 in 100 ml NS), and maximally dilute antivenin. Begin antivenin slowly. If needed begin epi drip at low dose [1 ml/hr of above mixture ~ 0.1 µg/kg/min] Once allergic reaction gone, restart antivenin slowly. Contact local poison center.

Elapidae (Coral Snake) Envenomation

This species is found in the southeast US and Arizona. They must bite and chew. Symptoms are primarily systemic and not local: altered mentation, cranial nerve or muscle weakness, respiratory failure. Symptoms may be delayed up to 24 h. Admit all for possible respiratory or neurologic deterioration. All require Coral Snake Antivenin. *Dose of antivenin:* 3-6 vials administered as crotalidae antivenin. Sonoran coral snake (also known as Arizona coral snake) venom is less toxic, no deaths have been reported, and coral snake antivenin is ineffective.

Special Situations

Mojave rattlesnake: May cause muscle weakness, paralysis, or respiratory failure with few local symptoms.   Crotalidae Polyvalent Immune Fab (Ovine) is effective, Antivenin Crotalidae Polyvalent is not.

Exotic snakes: Call **(602) 626-6016** for information regarding available anti-venin.

Serum sickness will develop in most receiving > 5 vials of antivenin within 5-20 days causing joint pain, myalgias, and possibly rash.   Warn patient and treat with diphenhydramine (*Benadryl*) 25-50 mg PO q4-6 h and prednisone 50 mg PO qd.

Spider Bites

Black Widow Spiders	Features of Black Widow Bites
• Found in all of US, mostly South	• Mild-moderate pain, redness, swelling, cramping at bite which later spreads
• Females average 5 cm with legs	• Abdominal wall pain mimics peritonitis
• Only females are toxic	• ↓BP, shock, coma, respiratory failure
• 1/5 have red hour glass on abdomen	

Management of Black Widow Spider Bites	Indications[1] for Admission/Antivenin
• Ca^{+2} gluconate 10%, 10 ml IV	• Respiratory or cardiac symptoms
• Lorazepam (*Ativan*) 1-3 mg IV	• Pregnancy or > 65 y with symptoms
• Consider Antivenin – Dose: 1-2 vials IV in 50-100 ml NS Skin test prior to using Allergy & serum sickness can occur	• Severe cramping or pain despite calcium and lorazepam use
	• History of ↑ BP or cardiac disease

[1]controversial   *Emerg Med Clin North Am* 1992; 269

Brown Recluse Spiders	Management
• Live mostly in southern US, and dark places. Bites are mild or painless.	• Wound care, tetanus
• At 1st lesions are red and blanch	• Consider referral to plastic surgeon for possible excision if > 2 cm & well-circumscribed border (usually 2 to 3 weeks after bite)
• Later a macule, ulcer or blister	
• Arthralgias, GI upset, DIC, or shock	
• Hemoglobinuria (renal failure)	• ± Dapsone 50-200 mg/day PO
	• ± Hyperbaric oxygen (controversial)

Marine Envenomation

↙ Puncture Wounds ↘

Sea snakes, blue ring octopus cone shells	Starfish, sea urchin, stingrays, catfish weeverfish, scorpionfish

↓

Lymphatic venous occlusion and pressure immobilization	• Immerse in hot water (45C) X 30-90 min or until pain subsides • Control pain with IV narcotics • Irrigate, after local/regional anesthesia • Debride + obtain xray to look for spine

↓

Supportive and respiratory care Sea snake antivenin[1,3]	Provide supportive care and administer Stone fish (scorpionfish) antivenin[2,3]

[1] *Sea snakes*. Bites are painless, causing paralysis + muscle necrosis. Administer polyvalent sea snake antivenin (Commonwealth Serum Lab, Australia) within 36 h. If unavailable, Tiger snake and polyvalent *Elapidae* antivenin are effective.

[2] *Stone fish (a type of scorpionfish)*. Venom causes muscle toxicity, with paralysis of cardiac, skeletal, and involuntary muscles. Pain is immediate and intense. The wound is ischemic, cyanotic and may lose tissue. Heat (45C) partially inactivates venom. Follow package insert for antivenin (Commonwealth Serum Labs, Australia).

[3] In US, call **(619) 222-6363** or **(415) 770-7171** for antivenin.

↙ Marine Exposures Causing Urticaria or Vesicles ↘

Hydroids, fire coral, jellyfish, anemones	Sponges, bristleworms

↓

• Apply acetic acid 5%, isopropyl alcohol, 40-70%, or baking soda x 30 min • Remove nematocysts with forceps[1]	Extract spicules, with adhesive tape

(right column) ↓

Acetic acid 5% or isopropyl alcohol

↓

• Supportive care if systemic reaction • Antivenin for box jellyfish, *C. flexneri* • Consider systemic steroids	• Topical steroids if mild reaction • Treat for allergic reactions

[1] Do not rinse in fresh water.

Marine Infections

- Organisms causing soft tissue infection: *Aeromonas hydrophilia, B. fragilis, E. coli, Pseudomonas, Salmonella, Vibrio, Staph./Strep. species, C. perfringens.*
- Irrigate, debride, explore, and obtain x-rays to exclude foreign bodies
- Antibiotic agents for treating soft tissue infection or prophylaxis:
  <u>Parenteral agents</u> - 3rd generation cephalosporin and/or an aminoglycoside
  <u>Oral agents</u> -Septra, doxycycline, cefuroxime, or ciprofloxacin

Gastrointestinal Bleeding

Diagnostic Evaluation of Upper GI Bleeding

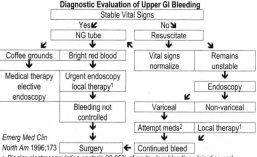

Emerg Med Clin North Am 1996;173

1 Bipolar electrocoagulation controls 90-95% of acute ulcer bleeding. Injection and sclerotherapy are effective against ulcers and variceal bleeding. Results differ depending upon site and magnitude of bleed.

2 Meds include (1) _Octreotide_ OR _Somatostatin_ – lowers portal venous pressure by splanchnic vasoconstriction. <u>Octreotide dose:</u> 50 μg bolus, then 50 μg/h IV. <u>Somatostatin dose:</u> 250 μg IV, then 250 μg/h. OR (2) Vasopressin (_Pitressin_) - <u>Dose:</u> Start 0.4 u/min, gradual increase to maximum 0.9 units/minute IV. Side effects: ↓BP, bowel ischemia, myocardial ischemia, skin necrosis. Nitroglycerin IV (40-400 ug/min) can limit these effects.

Upper GI Bleeding Etiology and Management

Resuscitation of Upper GI Bleeding	Etiology of UGI bleed - Admitted	
• O₂, cardiac monitor, insert NG, NS 2 L IV. Consider transfusion, FFP if unknown coagulopathy or PT or PTT > 1.5 X normal	Duodenal ulcer	36%
	Gastric ulcer	24%
	Varices and Gastritis (each)	6%
• Type & cross 4-6U PRBC's. Obtain CBC, platelets, electrolytes¹, LFTs, and PT/PTT. Obtain CXR and ECG.	Esophagitis/M.Weiss (each)	4%
	Gastroduodenitis	3%
	Other or source not found	17%
• Administer platelets if level is < 50,000/ml	_Am J Gastroenterol_ 1995: 208	

1 BUN/Cr ratio ≥ 36 indicates a > 95% likelihood the source of bleeding is upper GI.

UGI Bleed Mortality based on NG Aspirate (NGAsp) and Stool Color		
NG Asp	Stool color	Mortality
Clear	Brown or red	6%
Coffee	Brown/black	8.2%
Grounds	Red	19.1%
Red	Black	12.3%
Red	Brown	19.4%
Red	Red	28.7%
Gastroenterol Clin North Am 2000;29:275		

UGI Bleed Mortality Based on Number Diseased Organ Systems		
Number	Mortality	Systems
0	2.6%	Cardiac, CNS,
1-2	6-10%	Lung, Liver, GI,
3	14.6%	Renal, Major
4	27%	Physiologic
5	44.1%	Stress
6	66.7%%	
Emerg Med Clin North Am 1999;17: 239.		

Mortality Risk Score in Upper GI Bleeding

Component	Abbreviated Score				Total[1]	Mortality
	0	1	2	3	0	0-0.2%
Age	< 60	60-70	≥ 80	--	1	2.4-3%
HR and Systolic BP	< 100 & ≥ 100	> 100 & ≥ 100	> 100 & < 100	--	2	5.6%
Comorbidity	None	None	IHD[2], CHF[3], or any major disease	Organ[4] failure or cancer[5]	3	11-12.2%
					4	21-24.6%
					5	35-39.6%
					6 - 7	50-75%

[1]Add total points from abbreviated score. [2]IHD-ischemic heart disease, [3]Congestive heart failure, [4]Organ failure including renal or liver failure, [5]Cancer – disseminated malignancy
Lancet 1996; 347: 1138

Indications for ICU Admission in Upper GI Bleeding[1]	Indications for Surgery Consult in Upper GI Bleeding[1]
Hypotension or orthostasis	Variceal Bleeding
Hematochezia or hematemesis	Peptic ulcer with > 4 units transfused
Active GI bleeding	> 2 cm ulcer on endoscopy
2 or greater comorbidities	Endoscopy with stigmata of recent bleed
Significant coronary artery disease	Vascular malformation bleeding
Endoscopy-recent bleed, visible vessels	Aortoenteric fistula known or suspected
Onset or recurrence of bleed in hospital	Bowel perforation known or suspected
Multiple units of blood transfused	*Emerg Med Clin North Am 1996; 14: 523.*
Variceal bleeding	*Emerg Med Clin North Am 1999; 17: 239.*

[1]These lists are not absolute indications and clinical judgement must be applied.

Testing gastric aspirate for blood.

- Use gastroccult system to test for blood as hemoccult tests are inaccurate at low pH. Up to 20% with upper GI bleed have negative NG aspirates.
- <u>False positive hemoccult/gastroccult</u> occur with iron, red fruits, rare meat, iodine.
- <u>False negative hemoccult/gastroccult</u> occur with vitamin C, antacids, bile.

Lower GI Bleeding

Most common source of massive lower GI bleeding is an upper GI site, therefore all patients require NG tube. 80-90% of lower bleeding will stop without therapy.
Diverticulosis - 75% of bleeds are from right colon. Bleeding is arterial, and often massive. Pain is mild and crampy in nature. 50% rebleed & 20% require surgery.
Angiodysplasia - Acquired disorder of unknown cause. Lesions are usually in cecum and ascending colon. Barium studies and colonoscopy may not show these lesions. Selective mesenteric angiography is accurate.

Most Common Sources of Lower GI Bleeding[1]	
Diverticulosis	35%
Angiodysplasia	30%
Cancer polyps	10%
Rectal disease	7%
Other causes	3%
Undiagnosed	15%

[1]*excluding upper GI*

Assessment and Management of Lower GI Bleeding

Liver Disease

Liver Function Tests in Liver Disease[1,2]

Disease	AST/SGOT	ALT/SGPT	Alk phos	Bilirubin	Albumin
Abscess	1 – 4 X ↑	1 – 4 X ↑	1 – 3 X ↑	1 – 4 X ↑	Normal
Acetaminophen	50-100 X ↑	50-100 X ↑	1 – 2 X ↑	1 – 5 X ↑	Normal
Alcohol Hepatitis	AST>ALT - 2:1 (2 – 5X↑)		10 X ↑	1 – 5 X ↑	Chronic ↓
Biliary cirrhosis	1 – 2 X ↑	1 – 2 X ↑	1 – 4 X ↑	1 – 2 X ↑	↓
Chronic Hepatitis	1 – 20 X ↑	1 – 20 X ↑	1 – 3 X ↑	1 – 3 X ↑	↓
Viral Hepatitis	5 – 50 X ↑	5 – 50 X ↑	1 – 3 X ↑	1 – 3 X ↑	Normal

[1]Magnitude of test elevation above normal (10 X ↑), = 10 fold increase above normal
[2]Levels for different diseases can be variable, and numbers detailed are not absolutes.

Ascitic-Peritoneal Fluid Analysis

Disease	SACG[1]	WBCs – mm[3]	PMNs – mm[3]	Ascitic RBCs	Protein g/dl	Glucose mg/dl	LDH IU/L
Cardiac	> 1.1	~ 500	< 250	few	~ 4.0	~ 150	~ 100
Cirrhosis	> 1.1	< 500	< 250	few	~ 2.0	~ 130	½serum
LiverCa[2]	> 1.1	varies	varies	few	~ 2.0	~ 130	~ 150
Livermt[3]	> 1.1	~ 2000	~ 500	few	~ 2.0	~ 100	~ 200
Pancreas	< 1.1	~ 4000	~ 3000	few	~ 3.0	~ 200	~ 2000
Perfrtn[4]	varies	> 1000	> 250	varies	~ 2.5	< 50	~ 1000
Renal	< 1.1	< 500	< 250	few	~ 0.5	~ 100	½serum
SBP[5]	> 1.1	> 1000	> 250	few	~ 1.0	~ 130	~ 200
TB	varies	~ 500	~ 1000	high	~ 4.0	< 100	~ 300

[1]Ratio of serum to ascitic fluid albumin concentration, [2]hepatocellular carcinoma, [3]liver metastasis, [4]perforation of bowel, [5]spontaneous bacterial peritonitis.

Etiology of Ascites

Liver disease	78%	CHF	5%	Pancreas		1%
Cancer	12%	TB	2%	Renal, surgery, Chlamydia	< 1% each

Spontaneous Bacterial Peritonitis

Clinical Features				Organisms	
Ascites	100%	↓ LOC	51-54%	Gram (-) bacilli	72%
EtOH abuse	84%	Rebound	42-47%	Gram (+) cocci	29%
Temp >100F	54-68%	Asterixis	46-54%	Anaerobes	5%
Abd pain	51-79%	↓bowel sounds	21-54%	Miscellaneous	2%
Abd tender	51-79%	SBP < 90	5-14%	Polymicrobial	8%

See page 93 for antibiotic choice.

Hepatic Encephalopathy (HE)

Grade	Description
1	Irritable, slurring, asterixis
2	Lethargy, confusion
3	Somnolence, reacts to pain
4	Coma (↑ ICP)

Most common Precipitants of HE

Azotemia	26%	Alkalosis	7%
Drugs	24%	Infection	5%
GI bleed	20%	Constipation	5%
Protein use	7%	Other	6%

Management of Hepatic Encephalopathy

- Exclude precipitant/complication – *see above*, check glucose, manage ABC's
- ICU admit if grade II encephalopathy – see above. Intubate if grade III.
- Lactulose – 30-45 ml po tid/qid Or 300 ml via retention enema, low protein diet
- Neomycin 1-2 g/day po (or substitute vancomycin, or *Flagyl* due to toxicity)
- Determine eligibility for liver transplant

Anemia

Anemia Differential Diagnosis

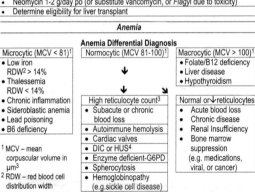

Microcytic (MCV < 81)[1]
- Low iron
  RDW[2] > 14%
- Thalessemia
  RDW < 14%
- Chronic inflammation
- Sideroblastic anemia
- Lead poisoning
- B6 deficiency

Normocytic (MCV 81-100)[1]

↓

↓   ↘

High reticulocyte count[3]
- Subacute or chronic blood loss
- Autoimmune hemolysis
- Cardiac valves
- DIC or HUS[4]
- Enzyme deficient-G6PD
- Spherocytosis
- Hemoglobinopathy (e.g.sickle cell disease)

Macrocytic (MCV > 100)[1]
- Folate/B12 deficiency
- Liver disease
- Hypothyroidism

Normal or ↓ reticulocytes
- Acute blood loss
- Chronic disease
- Renal Insufficiency
- Bone marrow suppression (e.g. medications, viral, or cancer)

[1] MCV – mean corpuscular volume in μm³
[2] RDW – red blood cell distribution width
[3] reticulocyte count X (Hct measured/Normal Hct)
[4] DIC – disseminated intravascular coagulation, HUS – hemolytic uremic syndrome

---

Sickle Cell Anemia

Diagnostic Studies in Sickle Cell Disease

- A routine Hb is recommended in most to assess severity or change of anemia.
- A white blood cell count often will be elevated due to sickle crisis alone.
- Obtain a CXR and pulse oximetry if cough, shortness of breath, or fever.
- Evaluate for crisis precipitant (e.g., infection, or dehydration).
- Consider a reticulocyte count if aplastic crisis suspected (Mean reticulocyte count for sickle cell patient is 12%, in aplastic crisis it may be <3-5%).
- Urine specific gravity is not a useful test for dehydration, as it may be low from isosthenuria (inability to concentrate urine).

Admission Criteria for Sickle Cell Disease

- Acute chest syndrome –pain/pulmonary infiltrate from infection or pulm. infarct
- Stroke, priapism, serious bacterial infection, aplastic crisis, hypoxia, acidosis
- Unable to take fluids orally or inadequate pain control in the ED
- Pregnancy, patients with uncertain diagnoses, persistently abnormal vital signs

Management of Sickle (SS) Cell Complications

Abdominal pain	• Patients with SS have ↑ risk for developing cholecystitis, mesenteric ischemia, or a perforated viscus. Splenic sequestration is rare in adults. Consider CT, ultrasound and surgical consultation (esp. if pain not typical of normal crisis).
Aplastic crisis	• Exclude reversible cause (medications) and transfuse for severe anemia (Hb < 6-7 g/dl) or cardiopulmonary distress.
Pain crisis	• Administer O_2 at 2-4 Liters. • IV ½NS at 150-200 ml/h (if mild pain, ± PO hydration) • IV narcotics titrated to pain relief (PO narcotics if mild pain)
Priapism	• Treat as pain crisis above. • Exchange transfusion to keep Hb S < 30% before surgery • Urology consultation for aspiration or alternate procedure.
Acute chest syndrome	• Admit all patients with a pulmonary infiltrate to the hospital. • Pulmonary infarct due to vaso-occlusion -may become infected. • Treat as pain crisis with IV antibiotics. Do not anti-coagulate. • Avoid angiography, as this procedure worsens sickling
Sepsis	• Admit all patients with invasive bacterial infections.
Sickle cell stroke	• Obtain CT ± spinal tap, Administer IV NS. • Exchange transfusion – keep HbS <30% total blood volume

---

Bleeding Disorders

Platelet and *capillary* disorders cause mucous membrane bleeds (GI, epistaxis, ↑ bleed with cuts, petechiae (↑bleeding time and abnormal platelets). *Coagulation* disorders cause hemorrhage of deep muscle, CNS, hemarthrosis, and ↑PT/PTT.

Factor VIII and IX Deficiency (Hemophilia A and B)
Severity of Bleeding and Dose of Factor VIII and IX

Severity	Specific Injury	Desired activity	Dose Factor 8	Dose Factor 9
Severe	CNS, GI bleed, major trauma, retroperitoneal or retropharyngeal bleed, pending surgery	80-100%	40-50 Units/kg	80-100 Units/kg
Moderate	Mild head trauma, deep muscle bleed, hip or groin injury, mouth or dental bleed, hematuria	40-50%	15-25 Units/kg	40-50 Units/kg
Mild	Laceration, common joint bleed, tissue or muscle bleed	20-40%	10-15 Units/kg	20-40 Units/kg

Replacement Factors and Medications used for Hemophilia

Medication	Dose
amino-caproic acid (*Amicar*)	• Primary use - to prepare for dental procedures • 100 mg/kg PO q 6 hours for 6 days
DDAVP *Desmo-pressin*	• 0.3 µg/kg in 50 ml NS IV over 30 minutes • Possibly effective via nasal spray or SC injection, recommended only if baseline activity > 10%
Factor VIII	• [desired activity level (%) – baseline activity level (%)] ÷2 • 1 unit/kg factor 8 will↑activity level 2% (T½ = 12 hours)[1]
Factor IX	• desired activity level (%) - baseline activity level (%) • 1 unit/kg factor 9 will↑activity level 1% (T½ = 24 hours) [1]
prednisone	• 2 mg/kg/day PO x 2 days is useful in mild hematuria

[1] T½ = half life and dosing frequency

Causes of Abnormal Bleeding Tests [1,2]

Lab Value	Causes
thrombocytopenia ↓ platelet count (<150,000/ml)	Heparin, ↓ platelet production, splenic sequestration, platelet destruction (drugs, collagen vascular disease, ITP, DIC, TTP, HUS)
platelet dysfunction (with normal count)	Adhesion defects (e.g. von Willibrand's disease) or aggregation defects (e.g. thrombasthenia), renal failure
↑ BT (>9 minutes)	All platelet disorders, DIC, ITP, uremia, liver failure, aspirin
↑ PTT (>35 sec)	Coagulation pathway defects (common factors 2, 5, 10, intrinsic 8, 9, 11, 12), DIC, liver failure, heparin
↑ PT (>12-13 sec)	Coagulation pathway defects (common factors 2, 5, 10, extrinsic 7) DIC, liver failure, warfarin
↑ TT (>8-10 sec)	DIC, liver failure or uremia, heparin
↓ fibrinogen,↑ FSP	ITP, liver failure, DIC

[1] BT-bleeding time, TT-Thrombin time, PTT-partial thromboplastin time, PT-prothrombin time, DIC-disseminated intravascular coagulopathy, ITP-idiopathic thrombocytopenic purpura, TTP-thrombotic thrombocytopenic purpura, HUS-hemolytic uremic syndrome.

[2] See pages 71, 72 for use and dosing of platelets, red blood cells, cryoprecipitate, and fresh frozen plasma

Managing Patients with High INR[1] Values[2, 3]

INR > therapeutic and < 5.0 and no significant bleeding	Lower the dose; or omit next dose. Resume therapy at a lower dose when INR is therapeutic. If the INR is only slightly above therapeutic, dose reduction may not be needed.
INR > 5.0 but < 9.0; no significant bleeding	(1) Omit next dose or two, monitor INR more frequently, & resume therapy at lower dose when INR is therapeutic. (2) Alternatively, omit a dose and give vitamin K_1 (1 to 2.5 mg orally) (esp. if patient is at increased risk for bleeding) (3) Patients requiring more rapid reversal before urgent surgery: vitamin K_1 (2 to 4 mg PO); if INR remains high at 24 h: an additional dose of vitamin K_1 (1 to 2 mg PO)
INR > 9.0; no significant bleeding	Omit warfarin; give vitamin K_1 (3 to 5 mg PO); closely monitor INR; if INR is not substantially reduced in 24-48 h, monitor INR more often, giving additional vitamin K_1, if necessary. Resume therapy at lower dose when INR is therapeutic.
INR > 20; serious bleeding	Omit warfarin; give vitamin K_1 (10 mg, slow IV infusion), supplemented with fresh plasma or prothrombin complex concentrate, depending on urgency; vitamin K_1 injections can be repeated every 12 h
Life-threatening bleeding	Omit warfarin; give prothrombin complex concentrate with vitamin K_1 (10 mg by slow IV infusion); repeat if necessary, depending on the INR

[1] INR – International Normalized Ratio

[2] If continuing warfarin therapy is indicated after high doses of vitamin K_1, heparin may be administered until the effects of vitamin K_1 are reversed and the patient becomes responsive to warfarin.

[3] Grade 2c – All recommendations are grade 2c which means (1) the risk to benefit ratio is unclear (2) supporting evidence is derived from observational studies and (3) the strength of the recommendation is very weak and other alternatives may be equally reasonable.

6th Am Coll Chest Phys Consensus Conference *Chest* 2001; 119: 22S-38S.

Management of Bleeding in the Dialysis Patient

- Direct pressure in bleeding from shunt (dialysis unit will have "shunt clamps")
- DDAVP 0.3 µg/kg in 50 ml NS IV over 30 minutes
- Consider protamine IV if recent dialysis

BLOOD PRODUCTS

	Cryoprecipitate
Features	• 1 bag (10 ml) has 50-100 units of factor 8 activity. There are 10 donors/bag. It has fibrinogen, von Willibrand's factor, factor 8 + 13.
Indications	• Hypofibrinogenemia if fibrinogen < 100 mg/dl. • Von Willebrand's (vW) disease & active bleeding - if DDAVP is unavailable or factor 8 concentrate with vW factor is unavailable. • Hemophilia A + unavailable monoclonal or viral inactivated factor 8 • Fibronectin replacement for healing in trauma, burns, or sepsis
Dose	• 2-4 bags for every 10 kg of bodyweight or 10-20 bags at a time

	Fresh frozen plasma (FFP)
Features	• Contains all coagulation factors. 40 ml/kg raises activity of any factor to 100%. This may cause fluid overload. ABO compatibility is mandatory although cross matching prior to transfusion is not.
Indications	• Coagulation protein deficiency if factor concentrates unavailable • Reversal of warfarin toxicity or active bleed with liver disease • Bleeding and coagulopathy with unknown cause
Dose	• If bleeding from vitamin K deficiency (liver disease) administer 10-25 ml/kg. 10-15 ml/kg will raise factor 8 levels 15-20%.

	Packed Red Blood Cells (PRBC's)
Features	• Fewer antigens are present in PRBC's compared to whole blood. • *Leukocyte poor* – use if transplant recipient or candidate, or 2 febrile non-hemolytic reaction • *Washed* – use if prior anaphylaxis due to IgA or other proteins. • *Frozen deglycerolized* - purest RBC product, use if reaction to washed RBC's or a transfusion reaction from Anti-IgA antibodies
Indications	• Acute hemorrhage or chronic anemia with hemoglobin < 7 g/dl • Symptomatic or underlying cardiopulmonary disease + Hb < 7 g/dl
Dose	• One unit raises hemoglobin by 1g/dl or hematocrit by 3%. • ≥ 2 units are needed in most circumstances.

	Platelet concentrate
Features	• 1 unit (pack) = 5-10,000 platelets. Platelets are not refrigerated & survive 7 days. ABO cross-match is not necessary, but preferred.
Indications	• Level < 10,000/μL unless antiplatelet antibodies • Level < 50,000/μL if major surgery, significant bleed, major trauma • Level - 10,000-50,000/μL if concurrent liver or renal disease that is causing platelet dysfunction
Dose	• 6 platelet packs (250-300 ml) or one plateletpheresis pack should raise platelet count by 50,000-60,000/uL.

BLOOD PRODUCTS continued

Whole blood

Features	• Has no WBC's and only 20% platelets after 24h. Factors 5 and 8 $\downarrow$60% and RBC's$\downarrow$ 30% after 21 days. With storage, K$^+$ and NH$_4$ $\uparrow$ (beware in liver failure) and Ca$^{+2}\downarrow$.
Indications	• Massive exsanguination, although this is better treated with PRBC's/crystalloid with replacement of specific components prn
Dose	• One unit contains 450-500 ml of whole blood

Transfusion Reactions
Crossmatching and ordering blood products:

• Type-specific non-crossmatched blood causes fatality in 1 in 30 million transfusions (most commonly due to labeling or patient identification error).
• Non-ABO antibodies occur in 0.04% of non-transfused and 0.3% of previously transfused.

Hemolytic transfusion reactions

• Occur in 1/40,000 transfusions and are usually due to ABO incompatibility.
• *Clinical Features* - palpitations, abdominal and back pain, syncope, and a sensation of doom. Consider in those with a temperature rise of $\geq$ 2C.
• *Management* - Immediately stop transfusion, and look for hemoglobinemia and hemoglobinuria. Perform direct antiglobulin (Coomb's test), haptoglobin, peripheral smear, serum bilirubin, and repeat antibody screen and crossmatch. Keep urine output at 100 ml/hour and consider alkalization of the urine to limit acute renal failure. Mannitol is not helpful, as it increases urine flow by decreasing tubular reabsorption without improving renal perfusion.

Anaphylactic reaction

• Almost exclusively occurs in those with Anti-IgA antibodies (1/70 people).
• *Clinical Features* - It usually begins after the first few ml of blood with afebrile flushing, wheezing, cramps, vomiting, diarrhea, and hypotension.
• *Management* - stop transfusion, treat with *Benadryl*, epinephrine & steroids.

Febrile non-hemolytic reactions

• *Clinical Features* - occurs during or soon after starting 3-4% of transfusions, most common if multiply transfused or multiparous with anti-leukocyte antibodies.
• *Management* - Stop transfusion and treat as transfusion reaction.

Urticarial reactions

• *Clinical Features* - causes local erythema, hives and itching.
• *Management* - Further evaluation unnecessary unless fever, chills, or other adverse effects are present. This is the only type of transfusion reaction in which the infusion can continue.

Hyperviscosity Syndrome

Etiology	Diagnosis
↑serum proteins with sludging & ↓ circulation. Common causes: macroglobulinemia, myeloma and CML.	• WBC (esp. blasts)>100,000 cells/mm^3 • ↑serum viscosity -Ostwald viscometer • Serum protein electrophoresis
Clinical Features	Management
• Fatigue, headache, somnolence • ↓vision, seizure, deafness, MI, CHF • Retinal bleed and exudates	• IV NS, plasmaphoresis • 2 unit phlebotomy with NS, and packed red blood cell replacement

Spinal Cord Compression

Most often due to lymphoma, lung, breast or prostate cancer. 68% are thoracic, 19% lumbosacral, and 15% cervical spine.

Clinical Features		Diagnosis
Back pain	95%	• Plain films are abnormal in 60-90%
Weakness (usually symmetric)	75%	• MRI or CT or myelography
Autonomic or sensory symptoms	50%	Management[1]
Inability to walk	50%	• Dexamethasone 25 mg IV q 6 hours
Flaccidity, hyporeflexia (early) or	-	• Radiation therapy
Spasticity, hyperreflexia (late)	-	• Surgery may be needed for epidural
Bowel/bladder incontinence	-	abscess/bleed, or disc herniation

[1] Steroid and radiation may be indicated if cancer is cause of compression.

Superior Vena Cava Syndrome

Occurs in 3-8% with lung cancer & lymphoma. Symptoms are due to venous hypertension in areas drained by superior vena cava. Death occurs from cerebral edema, airway compromise, or cardiac compromise.

Clinical Features		Diagnosis
Thoracic or neck vein distention	65%	• CXR shows mediastinal mass or parenchymal lung mass in 10%
Shortness of breath	50%	• CT is diagnostic
Tachypnea	40%	Management
Upper trunk or extremity edema	40%	• Furosemide 40 mg IV
Cough/dysphagia/chest pain	20%	• Methylprednisolone 1-2 mg/kg mg IV
Periorbital or facial edema	-	• Mediastinal radiation
Stoke's sign (tight shirt collar)	-	

Tumor Lysis Syndrome

Occurs within 1-2 days of starting chemotherapy or radiation for rapidly growing tumors (esp. leukemias and lymphomas).
Clinical features are due to hyperuricemia (renal failure), ↑K$^+$ (arrhythmias), ↑phosphate (renal failure), and ↓Ca^{+2} (cramping, tetany, confusion, seizures).

Management	Criteria for Hemodialysis
• Hydration with NS • Allopurinol 100-200 mg PO/day • Alkalinize serum with NaHCO$_3$ to urine pH ≥ 7.0 • Dialysis	• K$^+$ > 6 mEq/L • Creatinine > 10 mg/dl • Uric acid > 10 mg/dl • Symptomatic hypocalcemia • Serum phosphorus > 10 mg/dl

Hypertension (HTN)

Classification of HTN is based on measurements obtained on ≥ 2 physician visits.

Class	SBP/DBP[1]	Management[2,3]	If compelling indications[2,3]
Normal	< 120/80	Lifestyle modification for all classes	Renal disease, diabetes cut-off goal is < 130/80
PreHTN	120-139/80-89		
Stage 1 PreHTN	140-159/90-99	Thiazides for most, may consider [2] below	See drugs listed with underling disease risk below. Add second drug as needed.
Stage 2 HTN	160/100	2 drugs for most – thiazide and any from [2] below[4]	

Underlying disease risk	Diuretic	BB[2]	ACEI[2]	ARB[2]	CCB[2]	AldAnt[2]
Heart failure	+	+	+	+		+
Post myocardial infarct		+	+			+
High coronary risk	+	+	+		+	
Diabetes	+	+	+	+	+	
Chronic renal disease			+	+		
Prevent recurrent stroke	+		+			

[1] SBP systolic blood pressure in mm Hg; DBP-diastolic blood pressure in mm Hg; to classify, choose SBP or DBP that places patient into highest stage/class
[2] ACEI - angiotensin converting enzyme inhibitor, ARB - angiotensin receptor blocker, BB - beta-blocker, CCB - calcium channel blocker, AldAnt - aldosterone antagonist
[3] Routine tests before starting drugs: EKG, urinalysis, glucose, Hb, K+, Creatinine, lipids. Consider other tests if non-response to therapy or other disease suspected.
[4] Initiate combination therapy cautiously (esp. in those at risk for orthostatic hypotension)
7th Joint National Committee on Managing HTN

Hypertensive Urgencies & Emergencies

Hypertensive urgency - an elevated BP to level that may potentially be harmful if sustained (usually diastolic BP > 115 mm Hg) without end-organ damage.
Treatment goal is to reduce pressure gradually within 24-48 h to normal for patient.
The 7th Joint National Committee on HTN recommends
(1) combination oral antihypertensive therapy (see chart above),
(2) evaluation for heart or renal damage due to HTN,
(3) evaluation for reversible causes of HTN (e.g. non-compliance, sleep apnea, drug induced, chronic renal disease, renovascular disease, primary aldosteronism, chronic steroid use/Cushing's syndrome, coarctation of the aorta, pheochromocytoma, thyroid or parathyroid disease)

Causes of Resistant Hypertension

- *Improper measurement & Associated disorders* (obesity, excess alcohol use)
- *Volume overload*: excess sodium, renal disease, inadequate diuretic dose
- *Drugs/Other causes*: nonsteroidal anti-inflammatory drugs (esp. Cox 2 inhibitors), sympathomimetics (decongestants, anorectics, cocaine, amphetamines), oral contraceptives, adrenal steroids, cyclosporine, tacrolimus, erythropoietin, licorice, diet supplements (e.g. ephedra, ma haung, bitter orange)
- See reversible causes of HTN on page 74.

Oral Agents For Use in Hypertensive Urgencies

- Debate exists as to whether any acute treatment is needed in the ED setting.
- captopril (*Capoten*) - 25 mg PO bid/tid (administer 6.25 mg test dose if CHF). Onset is 30 min, peak effect 1-1.5 hours and duration 4-6 hours.
- clonidine (*Catapres*) - 0.1-0.2 mg PO. Repeat 0.1 mg PO q 1 h until diastolic BP < 115 mmHg or max. of 0.8 mg total. Onset 30-60 min, peak 2-4 hours, duration 6-8 hours. It is NOT necessary to initiate therapy with clonidine after ED use.
- nifedipine – can precipitously ↓ BP causing death. Do not use sublingual route.
- labetalol (*Normodyne*) - 100-200 mg PO. Onset is 15-30 min, peak is 1-3 hours, and duration is 8-12 hours.

Hypertensive Emergencies

- *Defined* - an elevated BP with end-organ damage or dysfunction. Treatment goal is to reduce MAP [Mean Arterial Pressure (MAP) = diastolic BP (DBP) + 1/3 pulse pressure (SBP-DBP)] by 20-25% in 30-60 min.
- *Catecholamine-induced hypertension* - Acute ↑catecholamines with acute sympathetic overactivity and hypertension due to pheochromocytomas, monoamine oxidase inhibitors, sympathomimetics, clonidine or β blocker withdrawal. Treat with labetalol or α-blockers (e.g. phentolamine).
- *Left ventricular failure and Coronary insufficiency* - ↑ afterload can lead to pulmonary edema, and myocardial ischemia. Nitroglycerin IV is the drug of choice. See page 39 for recommendations for treating acute pulmonary edema.
- *Hypertensive Encephalopathy* - headache, vomit, & confusion due to cerebral hyperperfusion with loss of cerebral blood flow autoregulation. Late: cerebral vasodilation, ↓blood flow, cerebral edema, papilledema, or exudates. Treat with sodium nitroprusside or labetalol (*Normodyne*). Lower MAP so CNS flow normalizes within 30-60 min. Do not lower MAP to < 120 mm Hg.
- *Pregnancy-induced Hypertension* or *Pre-eclampsia* - see page 117.
- *Renal failure* - ↓ renal function due to ↑ BP is a hypertensive emergency. Proteinuria, red cells, red cell casts and ↑ BUN/creatinine occur.
- *Thoracic dissection* – Treat with labetalol or (*Nipride* + esmolol). See page 40.

See Page 76 for choice/dosing of specific parenteral antihypertensive agents.

Drugs in Hypertensive Emergencies

Drug	Dose and route	Mechanism	Onset	Duration	Features
Enalapril (Vasotec)	1.25-5 mg IV over 5 min, administered q 6 h	ACE inhibitor	15 min	6 hours	Avoid in renal artery stenosis, useful if ↑ renin (scleroderma)
esmolol (Brevibloc)	500 µg/kg IV over 1st min, then titrate 50-200 µg/kg/min	β-blockade	seconds	half life = 9 min	Worsens bronchospasm, heart blocks, & congestive heart failure
fenoldopam (Corlopam)	0.1-1.6 µg/kg/min IV	Dopamine-1 receptor agonist	4 min	10 min	↑ renal flow, & Na⁺ excretion, esp. useful if ↓ renal function
hydralazine (Apresoline)	5-10 mg IV q 30-60 min or 10-50 mg IM	Arteriolar dilator	<30 min	4-12h	Causes tachycardia, headache
labatelol (Normodyne)	0.25 mg/kg IV, double q15min prn (Max = lesser of 300 mg or 2 mg/kg)	α and β blockade in 1:7 ratio	seconds	4-8h	Worsens bronchospasm, heart blocks, & congestive heart failure
nicardipine (Cardene)	Start @ 2-4 mg/h IV, ↑1-2 mg/h q15 min Max 15mg/h	Calcium channel blocker	1-5 min	20 min	Rarely precipitates angina, ↑HR and ↑ICP
nitroglycerin	5-200 µg/min	Vasodilator	2-5 min	5-10 min	May ↑heart rate, and ↓BP
propranolol (Inderal)	1 mg IV over 1 min q 5 min up to Max of 5-8 mg	β-blockade	seconds	up to 8h	Worsens bronchospasm, heart blocks, & CHF
phentolamine (Regitine)	2-10 mg IV q 5-15 min	α-blocker	1-2 min	30-60 min	tachycardia in pheochromocytoma
sodium nitroprusside (Nipride)	0.5-8 µg/min IV	Arterial and venous dilator	seconds	1-3 min	no ↓cardiac output, possible cyanide toxicity and ↑ICP

sec–seconds, min–minutes, h–hours, mo–months, mg–milligrams, µg–micrograms, PO–oral, SL–sublingual, IV–intravenous,

Occupational Exposure to Human Immunodeficiency Virus (HIV)

- Highest risk for transmission of HIV: (1) scalpel or needle visibly contaminated with patient's blood, (2) needle placed directly in vein or artery, (3) deep puncture or wound to health care worker (4) terminal illness in source patient.
- ZDV reduces transmission by ~ 79%. Begin prophylaxis ≤ 2-8 h from exposure.

Provisional Public Health Service Recommendations for Chemoprophylaxis after Occupational Exposure to HIV.

♦ Draw HIV, CBC, liver+renal function, βhCG ± hepatitis exposure work up (pg 78)

♦ Repeat CBC, liver/renal tests at 2 weeks, and HIV at 6 + 12 months

Exposure	Extent of Exposure	Source HIV + Class 1[1]	Source HIV + Class2[2]	Source HIV unknown
Percutaneous	Low severity[3]	Basic 2 drug regimen	Expanded 3 drug regimen	No prophylaxis[5]
	High severity[4]	Expanded 3 drug regimen	Expanded 3 drug regimen	No prophylaxis[5]
Mucous membrane/ nonintact skin exposure	Small volume[6]	*Consider* basic 2 drug regimen	Basic 2 drug regimen	No prophylaxis[5]
	Large volume[7]	Basic 2 drug regimen	Expanded 3 drug regimen	No prophylaxis[5]

[1] Class 1-asymptomatic HIV infection or known low viral load (<1500 RNA copies/ml)
[2] Class 2-symptomatic HIV infections, AIDS, acute seroconversion, or known high viral load
[3] Low severity-less severe; solid needle and superficial injury, [4] High severity-large-bore hollow needle, deep puncture, visible blood on device, or needle used in patient's artery/vein, [5] No prophylaxis generally warranted, consider if source has HIV risk factors. If source is later determined to be HIV-negative, prophylaxis should be discontinued, [6] Small volume-a few drops, [5] Large volume-major blood splash

Drug Regimens for HIV exposure (administer X 4 weeks)

Basic 2 drug regimen (all PO medications)	(1) ZDV (600 mg/day divided bid or tid) + 3TC (150 mg bid); aka combo product *Combivir* (1 tab bid) OR (2) 3TC (150 mg bid) + D4T (40 mg bid, if <60 kg decrease to 30 mg bid) OR (3) DDI (400 mg qd, if <60 kg decrease to 125 mg bid) + D4T (40 mg bid, if <60 kg
Expanded 3 drug regimen (all PO medications)	Basic 2 drug regimen AND one of following: Indinavir 800 mg q 8 or Nelfinavir 750 mg tid (or 1250 mg bid) or Efavirenz 600 mg qhs or Abacavir 300 mg tid (Abacavir is available in triple combination tablet with ZDV + 3TC as *Trizivir* 1 tab bid)

ZDV – Zidovudine, 3TC – Lamivudine, D4T, Stavudine, DDI - Didanosine

MMWR 2001; Vol 50/No. RR-11

Hepatitis B (HB) Exposure

Exposed Person	Source of Exposure		
	HB Surface (HBs) Antigen (Ag) positive	HB Surface (HBs) Antigen (Ag) positive	Source not known or not available
Unvaccinated	HBIG[1] x 1 and HB vaccine series[1]	Begin HB vaccine series[1]	Begin HB vaccine series[1]
Vaccinated *Known responder*[2]	No treatment	No treatment	No treatment
Vaccinated *Known non-responder*	HBIG[1] x 2 or HBIG[1] x 1 & initiate revaccination	No treatment	If high-risk source, treat as if source were HBs Ag positive
Vaccinated *Response unknown*	Test exposed for anti-HBs[2] (1) If adequate, no treatment. (2) If inadequate HBIG x 1 plus vaccine booster	No treatment	Test exposed person for Anti-HBs[2] (1) If OK, no treatment. (2) If inadequate, HB vaccine booster and recheck titer in 1-2 months.

[1] HBIG dose – 0.06 ml/kg IM, HB vaccine – 1 ml IM deltoid, repeat in 1 & 6 months
[2] Known responder - Adequate anti-HBs = ≥ 10 mIU/ml
Hepatitis A exposure: Administer ISG 0.02 ml/kg IM for exposure through close personal contact, employee at day care center, or contaminated food within 2 wks.

Tetanus Immunization

Prior immunization	Tetanus prone wound	Non tetanus prone wound
Uncertain or <3	dT, TIG[1]	dT
3 or more	dT if >5y since last dose	dT if >10y since last dose

[1] Tetanus immune globulin. Dose of TIG – 250 units IM at site other than for dT.

Postexposure Rabies Prophylaxis (*Ann Emerg Med* 1999; 33: 590.)

Rabies prophylaxis only indicated if bite or other salivary exposure from bat or carnivore. No prophylaxis is needed if nonsalivary or if bird, reptile, or rodent. If questions arise regarding prophylaxis and local and state health department unavailable call CDC at **404-639-1050** (days), **404-639-2888** (nights & weekends) (1) Rabies vaccine - 1 ml IM, on day 0, 3, 7, 14, & 28. Give in deltoid, not buttock. **PLUS** (2) RIG (rabies immune globulin) - 20 IU/kg infiltrated SC around wound (if possible) and remainder IM distal to site of vaccine administration.

		Animal is Cat or Dog	Not Cat or Dog
Was animal captured?	NO, escaped	Give RIG & vaccine only if rabies risk for species in area.	Treat with RIG and full course of vaccine.
	YES, captured	Observe animal for 10 days. If abnormal behavior, sacrifice and treat patient with RIG & vaccine. Discontinue treatment if animal pathology negative for rabies.	Sacrifice animal and begin RIG and vaccine. Discontinue treatment if pathology negative for rabies.

Acute Fever and Fever of Unknown Origin (FUO)

		Specific Infection/Etiology[1]	Frequency
Etiology of Acute Fever in IV Drug Users in the ED	•	Pneumonia	38%
	•	Viral, pharyngitis/bronchitis	21%
	•	Endocarditis	13%
	•	Pyrogen reaction or Unexplained	10%
	•	Cellulitis	5%
	•	Varicella or Tuberculosis	3% each
	•	Partially treated endocarditis, peritonitis, urinary infection, septic arthritis, osteomyelitis, GI bleed	3%
			2%
			1% each

1 No clinical data could exclude endocarditis, therefore admit all febrile IV drug users

Ann Intern Med 1987; 106: 823

		Specific Infection/Etiology[1]	Frequency
Etiology of Acute Fever in Patients ≥ 65 Years in the ED (Serious illness prevalence = 76%[1])	•	Pneumonia	25%
	•	Urinary Tract Infection	22%
	•	Sepsis/bacteremia	18%
	•	Unknown	11%
	•	Diverticulitis or colitis or cholecystitis	8%
	•	Bronchitis, pharyngitis or sinusitis	7%
	•	CHF, MI, stroke, or seizure	7%
	•	Cellulitis	5%
	•	PE, meningitis, prostate, cancer, GI bleed, dehydration, appendix, bone	1% or less each

Although fever ≥ 103F, RR ≥ 30, WBC ≥ 11,000, HR ≥ 120, and + CXR were associated with serious illness, 50% with none of these features had [1]*serious illness* defined as a positive blood culture, death, need for surgery, admit > 3 days, or ED visit in 72 h

Ann Emerg Med 1995; 26: 18.

		Specific Infection/Etiology[1]	Frequency
Etiology of Acute Fever in Nursing Home Patients	•	Urinary tract infection	34%
	•	Sinus, Pharynx, Upper respiratory	23%
	•	Skin	18%
	•	Pneumonia	8%
	•	Other (GI, CNS, bone, IV, multiple)	17%

Curr Clin Topic Infect Dis 1998; 18: 75.

	Specific Infection/Etiology[1]	< 65 years	≥ 65 years
Etiology of Fever of Unknown Etiology if < and ≥ 65 (fever ≥ 101F X 3 weeks undiagnosed after 1 week hospitalization)[1]	• Bacterial or viral infection	26%	36%
	• Multisystem disease	17%	28%
	• Tuberculosis	3%	10%
	• Abscess	4%	12%
	• Endocarditis	1%	7%
	• Tumor	5%	19%
	• Other/Unknown[2]	~ 40%	6%

[1] Recent authors have included patients with intensive unsuccessful outpatient evaluation
[2] Includes in decreasing order temporal arteritis, polymyalgia rheumatica, Wegener's granulomatosis, polyarteritis nodosa, rheumatoid arthritis, and sarcoidosis

Clin Infect Dis 2000; 31: 148.

Fever and Neutropenia

Fever – a single oral temp. ≥ 38.3°C (101°F) or ≥ 38.0°C (100.4°F) for ≥ 1 hour
Neutropenia – neutrophil count < 500 cells/mm³ or < 1000 cells/mm³ with a predicted decrease to < 500 cells/mm³

Clinical Score for Risk of Infection in Febrile Neutropenic Patients[1]			
Absent or mild symptoms	5	Solid tumor or no fungal infection	4
Moderate symptoms	3	No dehydration	3
Normal blood pressure	5	Outpatient onset of fever	3
Absent COPD	4	Age < 60 years	2

[1] Total ≥ 21 signifies < 10% probability of serious infection and potential to use less aggressive management options. *J Clin Oncol* 2000; 18: 3038.; *Clin Infect Dis* 2002; 730.

Empiric Antibiotic Choices in Febrile Neutropenic Adults

Low[1] Risk	Oral	• Cipro 750 mg PO bid AND Augmentin 875 mg PO bid
	IV Options	• Cefepime (*Maxipime*) 2 g IV q8h OR ceftazidime (*Fortaz*) 2 g IV q8h OR imipenem (*Primaxin*) 0.5-1.0 g IV q6-8h OR meropenem (*Merrem*) 1 g IV q8h.
High Risk[2,3]	IV Options (Mono or Combination Therapy)	• Monotherapy with cefepime, ceftazidime, imipenem, or meropenem (see IV dosing above) OR
		• Aminoglycoside [AG] (e.g. gentamicin or tobramycin 1.7 mg/kg IV q 8h or either AG at 5-7 mg/kg/d) PLUS one of: Timentin 3.1 g IV q4-6h, Zosyn 3.375-4.5 g IV q4-6h, cefepime, ceftazidime, imipenem, or meropenem (see IV dosing above)
	Vancomycin Regimen[2]	• Vancomycin 1 g IV q 12 h (max 2g/d) PLUS cefepime, ceftazidime, imipenem or meropenem (see IV option dosing)
		• ± aminoglycoside see dose under IV options above

[1] Only assign low risk and consider outpatient management if no bacterial infection is found, and closely coordinated follow up with hematologist/oncologist.
[2] Add vancomycin if suspect catheter related infection, colonization with penicillin and cephalosporin resistant pneumococci or methicillin resistant *S. aureus*, positive blood culture for gram positive bacteria before final identification and susceptibility testing, or hypotension or other evidence of cardiovascular impairment.
[3] If worsening course is expected and there is long expected delay in recovery of bone marrow, colony stimulating factors (e.g. filgrastim or sargramostim) may be helpful.

Fever and Rash

Causes of Petechial Rash and Fever

Infectious		Noninfectious
Endocarditis	Enterovirus	Allergy, thrombocytopenia
Meningococcemia	Dengue fever	Scurvy, Lupus
Gonococcemia	Hepatitis B	Henoch Schonlein purpura
Other pathogenic bacteria	Rubella, Epstein Barr	Hypersensitivity vasculitis
(e.g. Gram neg. enterics)	Rat bite fever	Rheumatic fever
Rickettsia (RMSF)	Epidemic typhus	Amyloidosis

Infect Dis Clin North Am 1996; 19: 101. & *Curr Clin Topic Infect Dis* 1995; 15: 19.

Causes of Maculopapular Rash and Fever

Infectious		Noninfectious
Typhoid fever/typhus	ParvovirusB19/5th disease	Allergy, serum sickness
Secondary syphilis, Lyme	Human herpesvirus 6	Erythema multiforme
Meningococcemia	Rubeola/Rubella/Arbovirus	Erythema marginatum
Mycoplasma, Psittacosis	Epstein Barr virus	Lupus, Dermatomyositis
Rickettsia, Leptospirosis	Adenovirus, Primary HIV	Sweet's syndrome
Ehrlichiosis, Enterovirus	Streptobacillus moniliformis	Acroderm. enteropathica

Infect Dis Clin North Am 1996; 19: 101. & *Curr Clin Topic Infect Dis* 1995; 15: 19.

Causes of Vesico-Bullous Rash and Fever

Infectious		Noninfectious
Staphylococcemia	Folliculitis (Staph,Candida	Allergy, Plant dermatitis
Gonococcemia, Rickettsia	Pseudomonas)	Eczema vaccinatum
Herpes/Varicella	Enterovirus, 5th disease	Erythema multiforme
Vibrio vulnificans	ParvovirusB19, HIV	bullosum

Infect Dis Clin North Am 1996; 19: 101. & *Curr Clin Topic Infect Dis* 1995; 15: 19.

Causes of Erythematous Rash and Fever

Infectious		Noninfectious
Staph/Strep infection	C. haemolyticum	Allergy, Vasodilation,
(toxic shock, scarlet fever)	Kawasaki's disease	Eczema, Psoriasis,
Ehrlichiosis	Enterovirus	Lymphoma, Pityriasis
Strep. viridans		rubra, Sezary syndrome

Infect Dis Clin North Am 1996; 19: 101. & *Curr Clin Topic Infect Dis* 1995; 15: 19.

Causes of Urticarial Rash and Fever

Infectious		Noninfectious
Mycoplasma	Adenovirus, Epstein Barr	Allergy
Lyme disease	Strongyloides, Trichinosis	Vasculitis
Enterovirus	Schistosomiasis,	Malignancy
HIV, Hepatitis B	Onchocerciasis, Loiasis	Idiopathic

Infect Dis Clin North Am 1996; 19: 101. & *Curr Clin Topic Infect Dis* 1995; 15: 19.

Human Immunodeficiency Virus

Correlation of HIV Associated Disease and CD4 Counts

CD4 cell count (mm³)	Infection or Other Complication
> 500	Acute retroviral syndrome associated with fever Candida vaginitis, Generalized lymphadenopathy
200 – 500	Sinusitis, bronchitis, bact. pneumonia (pneumococcus) Pulmonary tuberculosis (up to 40% have normal CXR) Herpes zoster, Candida esophagitis and thrush, Cryptosporidiosis, B-cell lymphoma
< 200	Pneumocystis carinii pneumonia, Disseminated herpes Toxoplasmosis, Cryptococcus, Histoplasmosis, and Coccidiodomycosis, Microspiridiosis, Tuberculosis (extrapulmonary and miliary), Kaposi's sarcoma
< 50	Disseminated CMV & *Mycobacterium avium* complex

Infect Dis Clin North Am 1996;10:149., *Med Clin North Am* 1996;80:1339.

Diagnostic Evaluation of Acute Fever in HIV

- **If localized signs or symptoms** evaluate & treat source
- **If central line, neutropenia, sepsis, IV drug use** – empiric IV antibiotics
- **If no local signs or symptoms** obtain following tests and (*manage as indicated*) - CXR/ABG (if *+treat for PCP, AFB, or fungi*), Urinalysis, CBC, LFTs (if + *US or CT abdomen and consider liver biopsy*), LDH (if + *with pulmonary symptoms treat PCP*), serum cryptococcal antigen, blood cultures (*culture for Mycobacteria & fungi*)
- **If above negative & CD4 < 200** consider (1) drug fever, (2) sputum/urine for TB (3) CT to exclude lymphoma (4) asymptomatic sinusitis – CT (5) dental source (6) spinal tap, (7) mycobacterial blood cultures (8) bone marrow

Infect Dis Clin North Am 1996; 10: 149.

	Specific Infection/Etiology	Frequency
Etiology of Acute Fever of Unknown Etiology in HIV patients (Fever > 100.4-101 F after 3 weeks if inpatient workup or 4 weeks if outpatient workup)	• Tuberculosis	5-42%
	• Mycobacterium avium complex	14-31%
	• Pneumocystis carinii pneumonia	2-13%
	• Visceral leishmaniasis	0-14%
	• Disseminated CMV, herpes/varicella	4-18%
	• Lymphoma	4-7%
	• Histoplasmosis or fungal	0-7%
	• Unknown	12%
	• Bacterial	2-5%
	• Toxoplasmosis or cryptosporidiosis	2-3%

Clin Infect Dis 1999; 28: 341. & 1995; 20: 872.

Meningitis
Typical Cerebrospinal Fluid Parameters

	Normal	Bacteria	Viral	Fungal	TB	Abscess
WBC/ml	0-5	> 1000[1]	< 1000	100-500	100-500	10-1000
%PMN	0-15	> 80[1]	< 50	< 50	< 50	< 50
%lymph	> 50	< 50	> 50	> 80	↑ Monos	varies
Glucose	45-65	< 40	45-65	30-45	30-45	45-60
Ratio[2]	0.6	< 0.4	0.6	< 0.4	< 0.4	0.6
Protein[3]	20-45	> 150	50-100	100-500	100-500	> 50
Pressure[4]	6-20	> 25-30	Variable	> 20	> 20	variable

1 – early meningitis may have lower numbers, 2 – CSF/blood glucose ratio,
3 – mg/dl, 4 - opening pressure in cm H_2O EM Reports 1998; 19:94.

Nomogram for Estimating Probability of Bacterial vs. Viral Meningitis

Severe Acute Respiratory Syndrome (SARS)

Visit: www.cdc.gov/ncidod/sars/ for updates re: evaluation/management SARS

Clinical Features of SARS

SARS - presentation	SARS Score[1]	
Incubation is 2-10 days. Early symptoms - fever, headache, and myalgias. By 2-7-days, a dry cough, shortness of breath are common with sore throat, rhinorrhea in < 10-25%. Xray confirmed pneumonia is found by 7-10 days in 97-100%. Diarrhea occurs in 73% Lab findings include	*Feature*	*Points*
	• Myalgias	1
	• Diarrhea	1
	• Cough during/before fever	-2
	• Rhinorrhea or sore throat	-1
	• Lymphocytes < 1,000/mm³	1
	• Platelets < 150,000/mm³	1

lymphocytes < 1000/mm³ in 70-95%, ↓LDH in 70-90%, ↓ platelets in 30-50%, ↑ PTT in 40-60%, ↑ CK in 30-40%, & ↑ ALT/AST in 20-30% and ↑ C-reactive protein.

[1] Total ≥ 1 was 93-100% sensitive and 71-86% specific in detecting SARS in 2 prospective studies of exposed febrile patients in Taiwan. An alternate study applied points to bilateral or multilobar pneumonia (3 points), < 1,000 lymphocytes/mm³ (2), SARS exposure (1), LDH > 450 U/L (1), C-reactive protein > 5 mg/dl (1), PTT > 40 sec. (1). Total alternate score ≥ 6 points was 100% sensitive and 93% specific for SARS

Ann Emerg Med 2004; 1, 17, 34.; *Emerg Infect Dis* 2004; 10:

CDC - Case Definition for SARS[1]

Clinical Criteria
Early: ≥ 2: fever, chills, rigors, myalgia, headache, diarrhea, sore throat, rhinorrhea
Mild-Moderate respiratory illness: Temp. > 100.4F/38C and one of following: cough, shortness of breath, or difficulty breathing
Severe respiratory illness: Mild to moderate criteria above AND one of following: Xray evidence of pneumonia, acute respiratory distress syndrome (ARDS), or autopsy findings consistent with pneumonia or ARDS without identifiable cause

Epidemiologic Criteria
Possible exposure to SARS associated coronavirus (SARS-CoV) with at least one of following: (1) travel to foreign or domestic locations with documented or suspected recent transmission of SARS-CoV or (2) close contact[2] with a person with mild to moderate or severe respiratory illness who has a history of travel in the 10 days before onset of symptoms to location with a documented or suspected SARS-CoV
Likely exposure to SARS-CoV – One or more of following exposures in the 10 days before onset of symptoms: (1) close contact[2] with a confirmed case or (2) close contact with a person with mild -moderate or severe illness for whom transmission can be linked to confirmed case of SARS-CoV in 10 days prior to symptom onset.

Laboratory Criteria
Serum antibody to SARS-CoV (turns positive 8-28 days after onset symptoms), isolation in cell culture from clinical specimen, or detection of SARS-CoV RNA by reverse transcription-PCR validated by CDC with subsequent confirmation.

[1] exclusion criteria - alternate diagnosis that explains SARS, negative SARS antibody > 28 days after symptom onset, or patient reported as suspected SARS due to close contact that was later determined not to have SARS

[2] cared for or lived with person with SARS or having high likelihood of direct contact with respiratory secretions or body fluids during period SARS patient was ill or within 10 days of symptom resolution.

Management of Suspected SARS Cases

- Isolation of respiratory tract and droplets (mask, gown, gloves, goggles for patient and medical personnel)
- Place patient in a negative pressure room.
- Screen all accompanying family and friends - see SARS CDC-Clinical Criteria listed on page 84.
- Initial diagnostic tests to consider include: Chest radiography, O_2 saturation, CBC/differential, LDH, Liver function tests, C-reactive protein, blood cultures, sputum gram stain & culture, Influenza A/B & RSV nasopharyngeal swabs, and urine antigens for Legionella, pneumococci.
- Acceptable lab samples include:
  1. Upper respiratory tract source: nasopharyngeal wash or aspirate, or swab, oropharyngeal swabs in viral transport media. Do not use calcium alginate or wooden swabs (these inactivate polymerase chain reaction tests - PCR)
  2. Lower respiratory tract source: bronchoalveolar lavage, tracheal aspirate, or pleural fluid in sterile container
  3. Blood: 5-10 ml blood in EDTA [purple top] & clotting tube for PCR testing
  4. Stool (> 10 ml) for PCR in dry container. Cool all samples to 4°C. Contact state/territorial lab/epidemiologist at one of the following email addresses for detail regarding case identification and appropriate laboratory testing and sample management.
  www.cste.org/members/state_and_territorial_epi.asp OR
  www.cdc.gov/ncidod/sars/lab/rtpcr/index.htm
- Treat with intravenous broad spectrum antibiotics in case superinfection or incorrect diagnosis and cover atypical causes of pneumonia.

Sepsis & SIRS

Systemic Inflammatory Response Syndrome/SIRS (≥ 2 of following)

• Temp > 38°C(100.4°F) or < 36°(96.8°)	• Heart rate > 90 beats/minute
• Resp rate > 20 or PaCO₂ < 32 mm Hg	• WBC > 12,000, < 4000 or > 10% bands

Early Goal Directed Therapy in Severe Sepsis and Septic Shock

Eligibility[1] - 2 of 4 SIRS criteria above AND
(Systolic BP ≤ 90 mm Hg after one 20-30 ml/kg NS challenge or lactate ≥ 4 mmol/L)

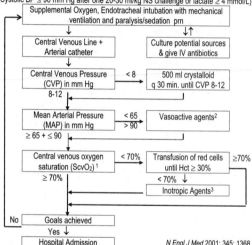

N Engl J Med 2001; 345: 1368.

[1]Original exclusion criteria (some are now relative contraindications) – age < 18 years, acute stroke, pulmonary edema, status asthmaticus, acute coronary syndrome, primary arrhythmia, active GI bleed, seizure, drug overdose, burn or trauma, uncured cancer, immunosuppressed, contraindication to central line, acute surgery needed, DNR status

[2] If MAP > 90 mm Hg, vasodilators are given to lower MAP to ≤ 90 mm Hg. If MAP < 65 mm Hg, vasopressors are given to maintain a MAP ≥ 65 mm Hg.

[3] Initiate dobutamine at 2.5 micrograms/kg/min. Increase dose by 2.5 micrograms/kg/min every 30 minutes until ScvO₂ is ≥ 70% or maximum dose of 20 micrograms/kg/min is given. Decrease dobutamine dose or discontinue if MAP < 65 mm Hg or heart rate > 120 beats/min.

Antimicrobial Therapy for Sepsis/SIRS

Possible Source	Antimicrobial Agents
UNKNOWN OR Immunocompromised	• [(Antipseudomonal Cp[3] or imipenem 0.5 mg IV q 6h or meropenem 1 g IV q 8h) plus (AG[1] or FQ[4])] OR • (Zosyn 4.5 g IV q 6h plus AG[1])
Abdominal	• See IDSA recommendations for intra-abdominal infections below
Abscess or Cellulitis	• (Imipenem 0.5 g IV q 6h OR meropenem 1 g IV q8h OR Zosyn 4.5 g IV q 6h) – ADD vancomycin 1 g IV q12 if methicillin resistant S. aureus suspected.
Necrotizing fasciitis, Gangrene	• Penicillin G 4 million units IV q4h OR imipenem 0.5-1.0 g IV q 6h OR meropenem 1 g IV q8h OR (Zosyn 4.5 g IV q6h + AG + Cleocin 600-900 mg IV q8h)
Pelvic - septic thrombophlebitis	• (Flagyl 1g IV) AND (antipseudomonal Cp[3], Unasyn 3g IV, Zosyn 4.5 g IV, OR Timentin 3.1)
Pneumonia	• See pneumonia page 93-95
Urinary	• ceftriaxone 1-2g IV q24h OR cefotaxime 1-2g IV/IM q12h OR FQ • If Pseudomonas (cefepime 2g IV q 12h or ceftazidime 1-2g IV q 8h) OR AG[1] OR FQ[4]
Wound or Vascular catheter	• Unknown/immunocompromised regimen above • AND vancomycin 1 g IV q12h

[1] AG – aminoglycoside (see dosing page 99-100); amikacin - least Pseudomonas resistance, tobramycin most intrinsic activity, & gentamicin - most Pseudomonas resistance.
[2] APP – Antipseudomonal penicillins (piperacillin 4-6 g IV q6-8h, ticarcillin 3-4 g IV q 4-6h);
[3] Cp – cephalosporins; Antipseudomonal Cps include – ceftazidime 2g IV q6h, cefoperazone 2-3 g IV q6h, cefepime 2 g IV q12
[4] FQ – fluoroquinolone. 2nd generation [effective vs. Chlamydia, Legionella, Mycoplasma, Pseudomonas, not strep]: lomefloxacin (Maxaquin), Noroxin, Floxin, [Cipro 400 mg IV q8-12h] 3rd generation – levofloxacin (Levaquin), (gram +activity), 4th generation moxifloxacin (Avelox), gemifloxacin (Factive), gatifloxacin (Tequin) [better anaerobic): [Cipro best anti-Pseudomonal activity)

Infect Dis Clin North Am 1999; 13: 495; *Med Clin North Am* 2000/2001

Infectious Disease Society of America Guidelines for Complicated[1] Intra-abdominal Infections

Severity	Antimicrobial Agents
Mild to Moderate	• Single agent regimen – Ampicillin/sulbactam[2] (Unasyn) 1.5-3.0 g IV q6h OR ticarcillin/clavulanic acid (Timentin) 3.1 g IV q4-6h OR ertapenem (Invanz) 1 g IM or IV q24h • Combination regimen – metronidazole (Flagyl) 15 mg/kg [max 1g] IV + 7.5 mg/kg [max 500mg] IV q6h] plus any one of: cefazolin 1-1.5 g IV q6h or cefuroxime 1.5 g IV q 6-8 h or Cipro 400 mg IV q 12h or (Levaquin 500mg,Avelox 400mg or Tequin 400mg IV q24h)
Severe	• Single agent regimen – piperacillin/tazobactam (Zosyn) 3.375-4.5 g IV q8h OR imipenem/cilastin (Primaxin) 0.5-1.0 g IV q6-8h OR meropenem (Merrem) 1 g IV q8h • Combination regimen – metronidazole (Flagyl) 15 mg/kg [max 1g] IV + 7.5 mg/kg [max 500mg] IV q6h] plus any one of: Cipro 400 mg IV q12h, or aztreonam (Azactam) 2 g IV q 8h, or ceftriaxone 1-2 g IV q24h or ceftazidime 2 g IV q8h or cefepime 2 g IV q12h

[1] Infections extending beyond hollow viscus into peritoneum with or without abscess
[2] Avoid ampicillin in areas with increasing E. coli resistance   *Clin Infect Dis* 2003; 37: 997

Therapy - Empiric Antimicrobial Coverage & Specific Infections in Adults[1]

Infection	Treatment
Abdomen	• See IDSA abdominal infection guidelines (pg 87)
Abortion – septic	• See chorioamnionitis page 89
Abscess	• In general, drainage required see specific site within text for antimicrobials (e.g. brain, breast, parapharyngeal)
Acne vulgaris	• Mild inflammation: tretinoin (Retin A) 0.025-0.1% cream gel qhs OR adapalene (Differin) 0.1% cream/gel qhs • Moderate: (Eryderm/Erygel 2-3% or Cleocin T gel bid) AND [benzoyl peroxide (Benzyl, Desquam) gel/cream qd-bid or Benzamycin Pak (erythromycin 3%+benzoyl peroxide 5% gel) bid or BenzaClin (benzoyl peroxide 5% + clindamycin 1% gel) • Severe: doxycycline 100 mg PO bid OR azithromycin pulse therapy (500 mg PO qd X 4days/month X 4 months) OR clindamycin 300-450 mg PO qid
Anthrax	• (Exposure and disease treatment) See page 10.
Appendicitis	• See IDSA abdominal infection guidelines (pg 87)
Balanitis - Candida	• See vaginitis Candida ± cover strep. or Trichomonas
Bite infection – dog or cat or rat	• Augmentin 875 mg PO bid X 10 d (1st line listed bites) OR cat – Ceftin 500 mg PO bid OR dog – Cleocin 300 mg PO q6h + FQ[2] OR rat/cat/dog – doxycycline 100 mg PO bid X 10 days
Bite infection - human	• Oral - Augmentin 875 mg PO bid OR (penicillin + cephalosporin) X 10-14 days (shorter if prophylaxis) • IV - Unasyn 3 g IV q6h OR Mefoxin 2 g IV q8h OR Timentin 3.1 g IV q6h OR Zosyn 3.375-4.5 g IV q8h OR Cleocin 600-900 mg IV q8h + Cipro 400 mg IV q12h
Botulism	• See biologic exposures page 11
Brain abscess	• Primary – (cefotaxime 2 g IV q 4h or ceftriaxone 2 g IV q12h) AND metronidazole (Flagyl) 7.5 mg/kg IV q6h • ADD vancomycin if related to trauma, surgery or recent admission (methicillin resistance suspected)
Breast abscess	• Lactating (S. aureus)– (nafcillin or oxacillin) 2 g IV q4 h OR cefazolin (Ancef) 1 g IV q8h • Not lactating (usually anaerobic) – Clindamycin 300 mg IV/PO q6h OR [lactating regimen above + metronidazole (Flagyl) 7.5 mg/kg q6h]
Breast infection	• See Mastitis page 91

Bronchitis – *see pg 131 for antibiotic indications*	• *Augmentin* 500-875 mg PO bid X 7-10 d **OR** *Zithromax* 500 mg PO qd X 3 **OR** *Biaxin* 500 mg PO bid X 7-14d **OR** *Biaxin XL* 1 g PO qd X 7 d **OR** FQ[2]
Brucellosis	• (Exposure and disease treatment) See page 11.
Cat scratch disease	• azithromycin 500 mg PO X 1, + 250 mg PO X 4d
Cellulitis – *uncomplicated healthy patient*	• Oral – dicloxacillin or *Keflex* 250-500 mg PO qid X 10d **OR** *Levaquin* 500 mg qd X 7-10 d, **OR** *Zithromax* 500 mg PO X1d, 250 mg PO X 4d **OR** *Biaxin* 500 mg PO bidX10d • IV – nafcillin1-1.5 g IV q 4-6 h **OR** *Ancef* 1 g IV q8h
Cellulitis – *diabetic, alcohol, (methicillin resistant S. aureus – MRSA)*	• Oral – *Augmentin* 875 mg PO bid **OR** IV/IM 3rd Cp[4] • IV mild-moderate– *Unasyn* 3 g IV q6h **OR** *Fortaz* 2g IV q8h **OR** cefoperazone 2 g IV q6h **OR** cefepime 2g IV q12: IV severe disease – imipenem 0.5-1 g IV q 6-8 h **OR** meropenem 1 g IV q8h. MRSA - linezolid (*Zyvox*) 600 mg IV/PO q 12 h. X 10-14 days.
Cellulitis – *lake/sea H2O (IV regimen differs if salt or fresh water etiology)*	• Oral: *Septra* 1 DS PO bid x 10 days **OR** FQ[2] x 10 days • If salt water – aminoglycoside (page 99) **AND** doxycycline 200 mg IV X 1, + 50-100 mg IV q 12h • If fresh water – ciprofloxacin 400 mg IV q 12 **OR** (ceftazidime 2 g IV q 8h **AND** gentamicin)
Chancroid	• azithromycin 1g PO X 1 **OR** ceftriaxone 250 mg IM X 1
Chlamydia – *urethritis, or simple cervicitis*	• azithromycin 1 g PO X 1 **OR** doxycycline 100 mg PO bid **OR** erythromycin 500 mg qid x 7-10d (treat gonorrhea)
Cholecystitis/cholangitis	• See abdominal infection choices page 87
Chorioamnionitis	• (*Mefoxin* 2g IV q6-8h **OR** *Unasyn* 3.0 g IV q6h **OR** *Zosyn* 3.375-4.5 g IV q8h) **AND** doxycycline 100 mg IV OVER 1-4h bid, switch to 100 mg PO when stable • **OR** *Cleocin* 600-900 mg IV q8h **AND** [ceftriaxone 1 g IV q12h or gentamicin (1.7 mg/kg IV q8h or 5 mg/kg/24h]
Clostridium difficile *diarrhea*	• *Flagyl* 500 mg PO tid X 10-14 d **OR** vancomycin 125 mg PO qid X 10-14 d • If cannot take PO: *Flagyl* 500 mg IV q6h ± vancomycin 1-3 ml/min of 500 mg/L saline solution per small bowel catheter or cecal catheter to maximum of 2g per day
Conjunctivitis	• *Ciloxan* 1-2 gtts q2h (while awake) X 2d, then q4h X 5 days. **OR** *Ocuflox* 2 gtts q2-4h X 2d, then 2 gtts qid X 5d **OR** (*Garamycin* or *Tobrex*) 1-2 gtts q2-4h or ointment applied bid-tid **OR** *Ilotycin* applied q2-4h
Corneal ulcer	• *Ciloxan* 2gtts q15 min X 6h, then q30min X 1d, then q1h X 1d, then q4h X 3-14d) **OR** *Ocuflox* 1-2 gtts q30min (while awake) X 2 days (awaken and instill q4-6h at night), then 1-2 gtts q1h X 5d, then 1-2gtts qid X 3d

Coxiella burnetii	• (Q fever evaluation & treatment) See page 12.
Dental infection	• <u>Oral therapy</u> - Augmentin 875 mg PO bid **OR** Cleocin 300-450 mg PO qid **OR** penicillin (↑resistance) 500 mg PO qid **OR** erythromycin 250-500 mg PO qid x 10 days • <u>IV therapy</u> – Cleocin 600 mg IV q6h **OR** Unasyn 1.5-3g IV q6h **OR** cefotetan 2g IV q12h
Diarrhea ...(*Salmonella, Shigella,* ...*Campylobacter, E.coli* or *Traveler's diarrhea*)	• Cipro 500 mg PO bid X 5 days **OR** Septra DS 1 PO bid X 5 days *(for severe symptoms – fever, bloody diarrhea)* – Only treat Salmonella if old, septic, immunocompromised, or ill enough to be hospitalized
Diarrhea *(Vibrio cholera)*	• Cipro 1 g PO X 1 **OR** doxycycline 300 mg PO X 1 **OR** tetracycline 500 mg PO qid X 3 days
Diverticulitis – outpatient	• *(Septra* DS 1 PO bid **OR** Cipro 500 mg PO bid) **AND** metronidazole 500 mg PO qid at least 7-10 days • **OR** Augmentin 500 mg PO tid X 7-10 days
Diverticulitis – inpatient	• See Infect. Disease Soc. America guidelines (page 87)
Ehrlichiosis	• doxycycline 100 mg PO bid X 7-14 days
Encephalitis	• See herpes encephalitis page 91, see biologic exposure to viral encephalitides (non-herpes) page 14
Endocarditis *IV drug use*	• nafcillin 2g IV q4h **AND** gentamicin 1mg/kg IV q8h
Endocarditis *native valve – empiric Rx*	• (penicillin G 20 mill units IV qd [continuous or divided q4h] **OR** Ampicillin 2g IV q4h) **AND** Nafcillin 2g IV q4h **AND** gentamicin 1mg/kg IV q8h • <u>Penicillin allergic</u> – vancomycin 15 mg/kg IV q12h **AND** gentamicin 1 mg/kg IV q8h
Endocarditis *Prosthetic valve empiric Rx*	• Vancomycin 15 mg/kg IV q12h (max 2 g/day) **AND** gentamicin 1 mg/kg IV q8h **AND** Rifampin 600 mg PO qd
Enterococcus faecium	• <u>Vancomycin resistant</u> – linezolid 600 mg IV/PO q 12h
Epididymitis – all ages	• Cipro 500 mg PO bid **OR** Floxin 300 mg PO bid X 14 d
Epididymitis ≤ 35 years	• see PID – outpatient treatment
Epiglottitis	• ceftriaxone (Rocephin) 2 g IV q24h **OR** cefuroxime (Zinacef) 0.75-1.5 g IV q8h **OR** Unasyn 3 g IV q6h
Francisella tularensis	• (tularemia exposure & treatment) See page 14.
Gangrene[5]	• *Gas gangrene, Fournier's, Necrotizing fasciitis* page 87.
Gingivitis – acute necrotizing, ulcerative	• Penicillin 250-500 mg PO qid **OR** tetracycline 250 mg PO qid **OR** doxycycline 100 mg PO bid X 10 days
Gonorrhea – *cervicitis, urethritis, pharyngitis, proctitis - Not invasive disease (PID, arthritis, etc)*	• <u>One dose PO of any of the following:</u> azithromycin 2 g, cefixime 400 mg, Cipro 500 mg, Floxin 400 mg, Tequin 400 mg, Maxaquin 400 mg, **OR** Rocephin 125 mg IM (also treat *Chlamydia* with azithromycin 1 g PO

Granuloma Inguinale	• See LGV treatment OR *Septra* DS 1 PO bid X 21 days
Helicobacter pylori	• (1) *Prevpac* as directed OR • (2) amoxicillin 1g and *Biaxin* 500 mg and omeprazole 20 mg PO bid X 14 d OR • (3) lansoprazole 30 mg PO bid and *Pepto Bismol* 2 PO qid + *Flagyl* 500 mg PO tid and tetracycline 500 mg PO qid X 14 d
Herpes - encephalitis	• acyclovir 10 mg/kg IV over 1 hour q8h X 2-3 weeks
Herpes – simplex Use oral agents and treat for half of *primary* time period if recurrent simplex	• Primary - acyclovir (*Zovirax*) 400 mg PO tid x 10 days OR valacyclovir (*Valtrex*) 1 g PO bid x 10 days • Labialis – recurrent – penciclovir (*Denavir*) apply topically q2h while awake for 4 days • Prophylaxis - acyclovir 400 mg PO bid OR famciclovir 250 mg PO bid OR valacyclovir 500 mg PO qd
Herpes - zoster if immunocompromised or ill consider IV therapy	• acyclovir 800 mg PO 5 x per day x 5-7 days • OR famciclovir 500 mg PO tid x 7 days • OR valacyclovir 1 g PO tid x 7 days
Impetigo	• Mupirocin topical tid ± see cellulitis page 89.
Influenza treatment (start within 48 hours of symptom onset)	• Influenza A or B: Oseltamivir (*Tamiflu*) 75 mg PO bid X 5 d OR zanamivir (*Relenza*) 2 puffs bid X 5 d OR influenza A only: rimantidine or amantadine 100 mg PO bid x 7d (100 mg qd if > 65 years)
Influenza prophylaxis	• Influenza A or B: Oseltamivir (*Tamiflu*) 75 mg PO qd X at least 7 d OR Influenza A: amantadine or rimantidine 100 mg PO qd X 7 days
IV catheter line infection	• Vancomycin 1g IV q12h If sepsis, immunocompromised or ill see Sepsis-Wound/Vascular catheter page 87
Ludwig's angina	• See submandibular abscess
Lyme disease	• See page 101.
Lymphogranuloma venereum (LGV)	• doxycycline 100 mg PO bid x 21 days • OR erythromycin 500 mg PO qid x 21 days
Mastitis (also see breast abscess page 89)	• Oral - dicloxacillin OR cephalexin 250-500 mg PO qid • IV - cefazolin 1g IV q8h
Mastoiditis	• cefotaxime 1g IV q4h OR ceftriaxone 1-2g IV q24h
Meningitis - bacterial < 50 years and healthy	• cefotaxime 2g IV q4-6h OR ceftriaxone 2g IV q12h • AND vancomycin 15 mg/kg IV q12h AND dexamethasone 0.15 mg/kg IV concurrent or 15 min pre-antibiotic and 0.15 mg/kg IV q6h X 4 days.

Meningitis – bacterial > 50 years or unhealthy	• < 50 year old regimen above **AND** ampicillin 2 g IV q4h • *Severe Penicillin allergy* –Septra 15-20 mg/kg/day (divided q 6-8 h) **AND** Vancocin 500-750 mg IV q6h
Meningitis exposure *(Neisseria meningitidis and Haemophilus influenzae)*	• *N. meningitidis exposure* –Rifampin 20 mg/kg PO q24h X 4 days (Max dose 600 mg) **OR** ceftriaxone 250 mg IM **OR** ciprofloxacin 500 mg X 1 in adults. Treat household, day care, or nursery contacts within 24h of case, older children/adults if kissed, shared food or drink or medical personnel exposed to secretions. • *H. influenzae exposure* - Rifampin 20 mg/kg PO q 24h X 4 days (Max dose 600 mg) if household contact when (1) household has unimmunized child < 4 years or immunocompromised child regardless of vaccine status (2) nursery or child care contacts when ≥ 2 cases of Hib invasive disease occurred within 60 days
Meningitis/ventriculitis ...CSF shunt or trauma	• <u>Shunt</u> - Vancomycin 1 g IV q 6-12h AND rifampin 600 mg PO q 24 h. Use ceftazidime (*Fortaz*) 2 g IV q8h if grams stain positive for gram negative bacilli • <u>Trauma</u> - Vancocin 1 g IV q6-12 + Fortaz 2 g IV q8h
Necrotizing fasciitis	• See Sepsis due to necrotizing fasciitis page 87.
Neutropenic fever	• See neutropenic fever guidelines page 80.
Oral-esophageal Candidiasis *immunocompromised*	• fluconazole (*Diflucan*) 200 mg PO/IV on day 1, then 100 mg PO/IV qd (oropharynx X 14 days or esophageal X 3 weeks & 2 weeks post symptoms) • itraconazole (*Sporanox*) oropharynx – 200 mg swish & swallow X 1-2 weeks or esophageal 100-200 mg swish & swallow X 3 weeks & 2 weeks post symptoms
Osteomyelitis - healthy	• nafcillin **OR** oxacillin 2g IV q4h **OR** cefazolin 2g IV q8h • If osteo from punctured rubber sole ceftazidime (*Fortaz*) 2 g IV q8h **OR** cefepime (*Maxipime*) 2 g IV q12h
Osteomyelitis – *if IV drug user, or dialysis, or immunocompromised*	• (Nafcillin or oxacillin 2 g IV q 4h or cefazolin 2 g IV q 8h) AND ciprofloxacin (*Cipro*) 200-400 mg IV q 12h • **OR** *Cipro* 200-400 mg IV q12h + *Vancocin* 1g IV q12h
Otitis externa	• *Cortisporin otic* 4 gtts qid **OR** *Cipro HC otic* 3 gtt bid X 7d **OR** *Floxin otic* 10 gtt bidX10d • <u>If severe</u> – dicloxacillin **OR** *Keflex* 500 mg PO qid **OR** diabetic regimen below. • <u>If diabetes (Pseudomonas)</u> – imipenem 0.5-1.0 g IV q6h **OR** meropenem 1 g IV q 8h **OR** *Cipro* 400 mg IV q12h **OR** ceftazidime (*Fortaz*) 2 g IV q8h **OR** anti-pseudomonal penicillin + aminoglycoside(pg99))

Otitis media	• *Amoxil* 250 mg PO tid **OR** *Augmentin* 500-875 mg PO bid **OR** cefdinir (*Omnicef*) 600 mg PO qd **OR** cefpodoxime (*Vantin*) 200 mg PO bid **OR** cefuroxime (*Ceftin*) 250 mg PO bid X 10 days
	• See otitis externa - diabetic if suspect *Pseudomonas*
Parapharyngeal abscess	• See submandibular abscess page 97
Parotitis – infectious	• Nafcillin or oxacillin 2 g IV q4 **OR** cefazolin (*Ancef*) 1 g IV q8h (ineffective if due to HIV, mumps, CMV, diabetes, mycobacteria, cirrhosis, malnutrition, medications)
Peritonitis – bowel perf.	• See abdominal infection recommendations page 87.
Peritonitis - spontaneous	• cefotaxime 2 g IV q8h **OR** *Unasyn* 3 g IV q6h **OR** *Timentin* 3.1 g IV q6h **OR** *Zosyn* 4.5 g IV q 8h
	• Resistant E.coli/Klebsiella (ESBL+[extended spectrum B lactamase +) Cipro 400 mg IV q12h or imipenem
Pelvic inflammatory disease (PID) – inpatient treatment	• (cefoxitin 2g IV q 6 h **OR** cefotetan 2g IV q12h) **AND** doxycycline 100 mg PO or IV q 12h x 14 days
	• **OR** *Cleocin* 900 mg IV q 8h **AND** gentamicin 1.5 mg/kg IV q8h. After discharge, doxycycline 100 mg PO bid ± *Cleocin* 450 mg PO qid x 14 days
PID – outpatient treatment	• (ceftriaxone 250 mg IM **AND** doxycycline 100 mg PO bid x 10-14 d) **OR**
	• ofloxacin (*Floxin*) 400 mg PO bid x 14 days **OR** levofloxacin (*Levaquin*) 500 mg PO qd X 14 days
	• ± ADD metronidazole (*Flagyl*) 500 mg PO bid x 14 days to either outpatient regimen listed
Pharyngitis *If group A strep. likely*	• Benzathine penicillin (*Bicillin LA*) 1.2 million units IM **OR** penicillin VK 500 mg PO bid **OR** cephalexin 250-500 mg PO qid x 10 days **OR** cefadroxil 0.5-1g PO qd x 10 days **OR** azithromycin 500 mg PO day 1, then 250 mg PO X 4 d **OR** clarithromycin 250 mg PO bid X 10 days
Plague	• (Exposure and disease treatment) See page 12.
Pneumonia – aspiration or lung abscess	• *Cleocin* 600-900 mg IV q8h **OR** cefoxitin 2g IV q 8h **OR** *Timentin* 3.1g IV q6h **OR** *Zosyn* 4.5g IV q 8h
Pneumonia – Influenza with mild bacterial superinfection *(in general requires admission)*	• (amoxicillin/clavulanate (*Augmentin*) 2 g PO tid or amoxicillin 1 g PO tid or cefpodoxime (*Vantin*) 200 mg PO bid or cefprozil (*Cefzil*) 500 mg PO bid or cefuroxime (*Ceftin*) 250-500 mg PO bid **OR**
	• [*Avelox* 400 mg PO qd or *Levaquin* 500 mg PO/IV qd or *Tequin* 400 mg PO qd or *Factive* 320 mg PO qd (each agent is given for 7 days)]

Pneumonia – Inpatient Medical ward admission Community Acquired (See PORT score page 133)	• [Avelox 400 mg PO/IV qd or Levaquin 750 mg PO qd or Tequin 400 mg PO/IV qd or Factive 320 mg PO qd (each agent is given for 7 days)] OR • [cefotaxime (Zinacef) 2 g IV q8h or ceftriaxone (Rocephin) 1 g IV q12-24h or ampicillin/sulbactam (Unasyn) 3 g IV q 6h or ertapenem (Invanz) 1 g IV q 24h AND [Zithromax 500 mg PO X1, then 250 mg PO qd X 4 or Biaxin XL 1 g PO qd Biaxin 500 mg PO bid X 7 days)
Pneumonia – Inpatient ICU admission Community Acquired (see PORT score page 133) *If Pseudomonas is NOT a concern* *(methicillin resistant S. aureus – MRSA)*	• [cefotaxime (Zinacef) 2 g IV q8h or ceftriaxone (Rocephin) 1 g IV q12-24h or ampicillin/sulbactam (Unasyn) 3 g IV q 6h or ertapenem (Invanz) 1 g IV q 24h AND • [Avelox 400 mg PO/IV qd or Levaquin 750 mg PO/IV qd or Tequin 400 mg PO/IV qd or Factive 320 mg PO qd (each agent is given for 7 days)] OR [Zithromax 500 mg PO X1, then 250 mg PO qd X 4 or Biaxin XL 1 g PO qd X 7 days or Biaxin 500 mg PO bid X 7 days) • If B lactam allergy – fluoroquinolone as listed above AND consider clindamycin (Cleocin) 600-900 mg IV q8h • MRSA – linezolid (Zyvox) 600 mg IV/PO q12h X 10-14 d
Pneumonia – Inpatient ICU admission Community Acquired (see PORT score page 133) *If Pseudomonas is a concern*	• [(Zosyn 4.5 g IV q 8h or imipenem 500 mg IV q6h or meropenem 1 g IV q8h or cefepime (Maxipime) 2 g IV q12h) AND ciprofloxacin 400 mg IV q 12h] OR • (Zosyn, imipenem, meropenem or cefepime as dosed above for ICU patients) AND aminoglycoside (AG6) AND Avelox, Levaquin, Tequin, Factive, Zithromax or Biaxin (see dosing above) • If B lactam allergy – aztreonam 1 g IV q 12h AND either Levaquin 500 mg PO/IV q 24 h alone or (Avelox 400 mg IV/PO q 24h or Tequin 400 mg PO/IV q24h plus aminoglycoside [AG6])
Pneumonia – Nursing home	• Treated in nursing home - [Avelox 400 mg PO qd or Levaquin 500 mg PO/IV qd or Tequin 400 mg PO qd or Factive 320 mg PO qd (each is given for 7 days)] OR [Augmentin 2 g PO tid AND (Zithromax 500 mg PO X1, then 250 mg PO qd X 4 or Biaxin XL 1 g PO qd X 7 days or Biaxin 500 mg PO bid X 7 days)] • Hospitalized – treat as per ward or ICU above.
Pneumonia – Outpatient *Healthy, No antibiotics past 3 months*	• Zithromax 500 mg PO X1, then 250 mg PO qd X 4 OR Biaxin XL 1 g PO qd X 7 days OR Biaxin 500 mg PO bid x 10-14 days OR doxycycline 100 mg x 14 DAYS

1-6 see page 99, PORT score – see page 133

Pneumonia – Outpatient (See PORT score page 133) *Healthy, Antibiotic use in past 3 months*	• *[Avelox* 400 mg PO qd or *Levaquin* 500 mg PO qd or *Tequin* 400 mg PO qd or *Factive* 320 mg PO PO qd (each agent is given for 7 days)]: **OR** • *(Zithromax* 500 mg PO X1, then 250 mg PO qd X 4 or *Biaxin XL* 1 g PO qd X 7 d days) **AND** (amoxicillin 1 g PO tid or amoxicillin/clavulanate (*Augmentin*) 2 g PO tid.
Pneumonia – Outpatient *(comorbidity – e.g. COPD, diabetes, renal or congestive heart failure, or cancer) NO antibiotics past 3 mo.*	• *(Zithromax* 500 mg PO X1, then 250 mg PO qd X 4 or *Biaxin XL* 1 g PO qd X 7 days or *Biaxin* 500 mg PO bid X 7 days) **OR** • *[Avelox* 400 mg PO qd or *Levaquin* 500 mg PO qd or *Tequin* 400 mg PO qd or *Factive* 320 mg PO qd (each agent is given for 7 days)]:
Pneumonia – Outpatient *(comorbidity – e.g. COPD, diabetes, renal or congestive heart failure, or cancer) Antibiotic use in past 3 months*	• *[Avelox* 400 mg PO qd or *Levaquin* 500 mg PO qd or *Tequin* 400 mg PO qd or *Factive* 320 mg PO qd (each agent is given for 7 days)] **OR** • *(Zithromax* 500 mg PO X1, then 250 mg PO qd X 4 or *Biaxin XL* 1 g PO qd X 7 days or *Biaxin* 500 mg PO bid X 7 days) **AND** (amoxicillin/clavulanate (*Augmentin*) 2 g PO tid or amoxicillin 1 g PO tid or cefpodoxime (*Vantin*) 200 mg PO bid or cefprozil (*Cefzil*) 500 mg PO bid or cefuroxime (*Ceftin*) 250-500 mg PO bid
Pneumonia – *Pneumocystis carinii*	• *Septra DS* 2 PO q 8h **OR** IV *Septra* - 15 mg/kg of TMP if ill q8h X 21 days • **OR** [(*Cleocin* 600 mg IV q8h or 300-450 mg PO qid) and primaquine 15-30 mg of base PO qd X 21 days] • **OR** pentamidine (*Pentam*) 4 mg/kg IV q24x X 21 days • **OR** dapsone 100 mg PO qd and trimethoprim (*Primsol*) 5 mg/kg PO tid X 21 days • **OR** atovaquone 750 mg PO bid X 21 days • **ADD** prednisone taper for 2-3 weeks if pO$_2$ < 70 mm Hg
Prostatitis ≤ 35 years	• see PID - outpatient treatment
Prostatitis > 35 years	• *Cipro* 500 mg PO bid x 14d **OR** *Septra* 1DS PO bid x 14d **OR** see epididymitis-all ages • Chronic prostatitis – may require 4 weeks of treatment

[1-6] see page 99, PORT score – see page 13

Pyelonephritis – *healthy*	• <u>Oral X 7 days</u>: *Cipro* 250 mg bid, *Levaquin* 250-500 mg qd, *Floxin* 200-400 mg bid, *Maxaquin* 400 mg qd, *Tequin* 200-400 mg qd, *Avelox* 400 mg qd • **OR** *Septra* DS mg PO bid, or oral cephalosporin (see dosing for UTI pregnancy) each for 14 days • <u>IV</u> (ampicillin 2 g IV q4h **AND** gentamicin [pg 99]) **OR** *Cipro/Levaquin/Tequin* IV (highest PO dose IV) **OR** *Claforan* 1g IV q12h **OR** *Rocephin* 1g IV qd **OR** *Timentin* 3.1g IV q6h, **OR** *Zosyn* 3.375-4.5mg IV q6-8h • If pregnant use IV *Claforan* or *Rocephin* as listed above
Pyelonephritis – *nursing home or Foley catheter*	• ampicillin 2 g IV q4h **AND** gentamicin [page 99] • **OR** IV fluoroquinolone-healthy pyelonephritis dose **OR** *Timentin* 3.1 g IV q8h **OR** *Zosyn* 4.5 g IV a 8h **OR** imipenem 0.5-1g IV q6-8h **OR** meropenem 0.5-1g IVq8h
Q fever	• (Exposure and disease treatment) See page 12.
Retropharyngeal abscess	• See submandibular abscess page 97.
Scabies (& head lice)	• permethrin 5% (*Elimite*) or 1% (*Nix*) <u>scabies</u> - massage cream into body & remove in 8-14 h, or apply lotion for <u>scalp lice</u> infestation (to dry hair) saturate for 10 min then rinse **OR** (*Eurax*) <u>scabies</u> - apply crotamiton (*Eurax*) <u>scabies</u> - apply chin down, repeat in 24 h, wash off in 48 h **OR** lindane (*Kwell*) <u>scabies</u> – apply lotion neck down, wash off in 8-12 h; <u>lice</u> – apply lotion or cream to affected areas wash off in 12 h, or shampoo with 30-60 ml lotion & remove in 4 min. **OR** ivermectin (*Stromectol*) 200 µg/kg (tabs are 3 or 6 mg) PO **OR** malathion 0.5% lotion – <u>lice</u> -apply to dry hair, dry naturally, wash off in 8-12 h, repeat in 7-9 d
Sepsis	*See page 87 for suspected source and treatment* • Drotrecogin alfa/recombinant human activated protein C 24 µg/kg/h X 96h if ≥ 3 SIRS features (page 86) & evidence sepsis induced organ dysfunction > 24h (preliminary data shows benefit/*New Engl J Med* 2001;March)
Septic arthritis (no trauma or operation)	• (nafcillin **OR** oxacillin 2 g IV q4h) **AND** (antipseudomonal Cp - see pg 99 **OR** *Cipro* 400 mg IV bid) • If suspect gonorrhea: 3rd generation cephalosporin
Septic arthritis (post trauma/surgery or prosthetic joint)	• vancomycin 1 g IV q 12h **AND** [*Cipro* 400 mg IV q12h or gentamicin 1.7 mg/kg IV q8h or aztreonam 1 g IV q8h or antipseudomonal cephalosporin IV]

Septic bursitis	• <u>IV therapy</u>: nafcillin OR oxacillin 2 g IV q4h OR *Ancef* 2 g IV q8h OR Vancomycin 1g IV q12h
	• <u>PO therapy</u>: dicloxacillin 500 mg PO qid OR ciprofloxacin 750 mg PO bid + rifampin 300 mg PO bid
Sinusitis	• <u>Mild disease</u>: treat as Otitis Media (pg 93); <u>Severe disease</u> (if well enough for outpatient treatment): *Avelox* 400 mg PO qd X 10 days, OR *Levaquin* 500 mg PO qd X 10-14 d, OR *Tequin* 400 mg PO qd X 10 d
Smallpox	• See page 13.
Submandibular abscess (surgery often required)	• Clindamycin (*Cleocin*) 600-900 mg IV q8h OR cefoxitin (*Mefoxin*) 2 g IV q8h OR *Unasyn* 1.5-3.0 g IV q8h OR *Timentin* 3.1 g IV q4-6h OR *Zosyn* 3.375-4.5 g IV q6h.
Syphilis – primary or secondary < 1 year	• benzathine penicillin (*Bicillin LA*) 2.4 million Units IM OR doxycycline 100 mg PO bid x 14d
Syphilis – secondary >1 year	• benzathine penicillin (*Bicillin LA*) 2.4 million Units IM q week X 3 OR doxycycline 100 mg PO bid x 28 days
Tinea - capitis & barbae (scalp & beard)	• terbinafine (*Lamisil*) 250 mg qd X 4-8 weeks OR griseofulvin (*Grifulvin V*) 500 mg PO qd X 6 weeks OR itraconazole (*Sporanox*) 3-5 mg/kg/day PO qd X 6 weeks OR fluconazole (*Diflucan*) 8 mg/kg q week X 8-12 weeks [max 150 mg/week] (**non-FDA recommendations** *J Am Acad Derm* 1999;40:S27) • **ADD** ketoconazole 2% or selenium sulfide shampoo
Tinea - corporis, cruris, pedis (skin, inguinal, feet) *Am Fam Physician* 1998; 58: 163 & *J Am Acad Derm* 1999; 40: S31-34. (not all oral agents are FDA approved for these indications)	• <u>Topical options</u>- ciclopirox (*Loprox*) bid, clotrimazole (*Lotrimin*) bid, econazole (*Spectazole*) qd, miconazole (*Micatin*) bid, naftine (*Naftil*) cream/bid, oxiconazole (*Oxistat*) qd, terbinafine (*Lamisil*) bid, tolnaftate • <u>Unresponsive to topicals</u>–fluconazole (*Diflucan*) 150 mg/week X 2-4 weeks OR terbinafine (*Lamisil*) 250 mg PO qd X 2 weeks (longer regimen for tinea pedis) OR ketoconazole (*Nizoral*) 200 mg PO qd X 4 weeks OR griseofulvin 500 mg PO qd X 4-6 weeks
Tinea ungium – nails & onychomycosis (not all orals are FDA approved for this indication) *J Am Acad Derm* 1999; 40: S21	• terbinafine (*Lamisil*) 250 mg PO qd X 6 weeks or pulse 500 mg PO qd X 1 week on/3 weeks off X 2 mo (use longer regimen for toes, shorter for fingers) OR fluconazole (*Diflucan*) 150-300 mg/week X ≥ 3 mo OR itraconazole (*Sporanox*) 200 mg PO qd X 3 ml or pulse 200 mg PO bid X 1 week on/3 weeks off X 2-3 mo

Tinea versicolor	• Topical options– ciclopirox (*Loprox*) bid, clotrimazole (*Lotrimin*) bid, econazole (*Spectazole*) qd, ketoconazole (*Nizoral*) – qd, miconazole (*Micatin*) bid, oxiconazole (*Oxistat*) qd, terbinafine (*Lamisil*) bid • Orals – ketoconazole (*Nizoral*) 400 mg PO X 1 pill or 200 mg/day X 7 days, OR fluconazole (*Diflucan*) 400 mg PO X 1 pill
Toxic Shock syndrome	• See page 102
Trichomonas	• metronidazole 2 g PO x 1 pill OR 500 mg PO bid x 7 days
Tularemia	• (Exposure and disease treatment) See page 14.
Urinary tract infection *Healthy, females, non-recurrent. If pyelo- nephritis see page 96*	• Simple UTI 3 days PO of any of following (if complicated outpatient use for 10-14 days): - *Septra* 1 DS bid, *Cipro* 250 mg bid, *Cipro XR* 500 mg PO qd, *Levaquin* 250 mg qd, *Maxaquin* 400 mg qd, *Noroxin* 400 mg bid, *Floxin* 200-300 mg bid, *Tequin* 200-400 mg qd
Urinary tract infection *Pregnant & Uncomplicated without pyelonephritis OR Pregnant asymptomatic bacturia*	• **Treat** 7-10 days for simple infection OR 3 days for asymptomatic bacturia - choose one of following: • nitrofurantoin (*Macrodantin*) 50-100 mg PO qid OR *Macrobid* 100 mg PO bid OR cefadroxil (*Duricef*) 1 g PO bid OR cephalexin (*Keflex*) 500 mg PO bid OR cefuroxime (*Ceftin*) 125-250 mg PO bid OR loracarbef (*Lorabid*) 200 mg PO bid OR cefixime 400 mg PO qd OR cefpodoxime (*Vantin*) 100 mg PO bid
Vaginosis, bacterial	• Oral - Flagyl 500 mg OR Cleocin 300 mg PO bid x 7 d • Intravaginal - metronidazole gel 1-2 x per day x 5 days OR clindamycin vaginal cream qhs X 7 days
Vaginitis - Candida	• miconazole topically bid X 2 weeks OR fluconazole (*Diflucan*) 150 mg PO X 1 dose OR itraconazole(*Sporonox*) 200 mg PO bid X 1 d
Herpes - varicella	• acyclovir 800 mg PO qid x 5 days (use IV dosing if immunocompromised, pneumonia or 3rd trimester pregnancy)
Vascular infection	• vancomycin 1 g IV q 12 h (*e.g.* IV, central line, dialysis)
Viral encephalitis	• See herpes, or see viral encephalidites page 14
Viral hemorrhagic fever	• (Marburg, Yellow fever, Ebola) See page 14

Warts	• <u>Anogenital</u> – imiquimod (*Aldara*) apply 3X/week qhs until clear (max 16 weeks) – wash off in 6-10 hours **OR** podofilox (*Condylox*) apply bid for 3 consecutive days/week, continue X 4 weeks (only apply 3 days/week) **OR** physician applied podophyllin 25% applied to wart for 30 min 1st treatment, then minimum time for desired result (1-4h) q week **OR** <u>Other therapy</u> by MD cryo-therapy, laser, trichloroacetic acid, bleomycin, surgery • <u>Cutaneous</u> – (1) topical salicylic acid (*Dr. Scholl's/Duo-Film/Clear Away wart remover*) bid or q48h if plaster or pad application X 4-12 weeks (over the counter) (2) tretinoin gel (*Retin A*) 0.025-0.1% topically qhs for verruca plana (flat warts) or (3) other therapy above.
Yellow fever	• See page 14 (viral hemorrhagic fever).
Yersinia pestis	• (Plague exposure/ treatment) See page 12.

1 The decision to use IV or PO regimens is complex. Listed medications are only recommendations. Consult textbooks, recent literature, and experts if uncertain about proper treatment options. Certain disease (e.g. fasciitis, gangrene, septic arthritis, osteomyelitis) may require surgical treatment. Drug doses may need to be changed or selections altered depending on cultures, renal function, & underlying disease.

2 FQ – fluoroquinolone (e.g. ciprofloxacin [*Cipro*] 250-500 mg PO bid, gatifloxacin [*Tequin*] 400 mg qd, levofloxacin [*Levaquin*] 250-500 mg PO qd, moxifloxacin [*Avelox*], ofloxacin [*Floxin*] 200-400 PO bid, sparfloxacin [*Zagam*] 400 mg PO day1, then 200 mg PO qd)

3 Macrolides – azithromycin (*Zithromax*) 500 mg PO X1, 250 mg PO days 2-5; clarithromycin (*Biaxin*) 250-500 mg PO bid x 7-10 d, erythromycin 250-500 mg PO qid X7-10 d

4 3rd Cp – 3rd generation cephalosporins (e.g. cefotaxime, cefizoxime, ceftriaxone)

5 Gas gangrene, necrotizing fasciitis, Fournier's gangrene, and Meleney's synergistic gangrene require similar antibiotics and surgical debridement. Consider hyperbaric O_2.

6 AG – aminoglycoside - amikacin - least *Pseudomonas* resistance, tobramycin most intrinsic activity, & gentamicin - most *Pseudomonas* resistance.

Aminoglycoside Dosing with Normal Renal Function[1,2]

amikacin (*Amikin*)	15 mg/kg/d IV divide q8-12h, max dose 1500mg/d.
gentamicin (*Garamycin*)	1.7 mg/kg IV/IM q8h, or 5mg/kg/d
tobramycin (*Nebcin*)	1.7 mg/kg IV/IM q 8h,

1 Gentamicin and tobramycin can be given once/day at 5-7 mg/kg IV q 24 h or amikacin can be given at 15 mg/kg q 24h. Administer over 60 min to avoid neuromuscular blockade. Draw level 8-12 h after starting infusion. Level is plotted on once daily algorithm & interval (not dose) is adjusted for subsequent doses.Endotoxin reactions reported with this regimen

2 Adjust aminoglycoside dosing regimen so peak serum levels (drawn 30 min after start of a 30-60min infusion or 60 min after IM injection) are sufficiently high to be bacter-

Drug	Peak	Trough
amikacin	15-30 µg/ml	< 5-10 µg/ml
gentamicin	6-12 µg/ml	< 2 µg/ml
tobramycin	6-12 µg/ml	< 2 µg/ml

icidal (see *peak* and below trough levels drawn 30 min prior to next dose).

Aminoglycoside Dosing in Renal Failure

- **Loading dose** – Administer the same loading dose regardless of renal function.
- *Estimate creatinine clearance* $CLcr = \dfrac{[140 - age\ (years)] \times weight\ (kg)}{serum\ creatinine\ (mg/dl) \times 72}$
- Multiply above X 0.85 for women

Maintenance dose for Traditional Dosing based on Creatinine Clearance

Creatinine clearance	Dose to administer OR interval alteration
> 50 ml/minute	• Administer 60-90% of traditional dose q 8-12 hours **OR** • Increase interval alone to q 12-24 hours
10-50 ml/min	• Administer 30-70% of traditional dose q 12 hours **OR** • Increase interval alone to q 24-48 hours
< 10 ml/min	• Administer 20-30% of traditional dose q 24-48 hours **OR** • Increase interval alone to q 48-72 hours

Maintenance dose for once daily aminoglycosides, alter 1st maintenance dose timing

Creatinine clearance	Timing of maintenance dose (gentamicin example given)
> 60 ml/min	Normal time for recommended interval (q 24h for gentamicin)
40-59 ml/min	At 1.5 X recommended dosing interval (q 36h for gentamicin)
20-39 ml/min	At 2.0 X recommended dosing interval (q 48h for gentamicin)
* Check 12 h level with this regimen. For **subsequent** doses, if 12 h gentamicin or tobramycin level is ≤ 3ug/ml widen the dosing interval to q 24 h, if 3-5 ug/ml administer q 36h if, 5-7 ug/ml administer q 48 h	

Differentiation Between Genital Ulcers[1] (see pages 89-97 for treatment)

Disease	Ulcer Description	Incubation	Painful	Inguinal Nodes
Syphilis	Indurated, nonclean base, heals on own	≥ 2 weeks	No	Firm, rubbery, tender nodes (painless ulcer)
Herpes simplex	Multiple, small grouped vesicles or ulcers with scalloped borders	2-7 d	Yes	Tender, bilateral lymph nodes
Chancroid	Irregular purulent, undermined edges, no induration, occasionally multiple	2-12 days	Yes	Very painful, fluctuant, craters may form, unilocular
Lympho-granuloma venereum	Usually not observed, small and shallow, often heal spontaneously	5-21 days	No	Matted clusters of nodes, unilateral or bi-lateral, multiloculated.
	May be above and below inguinal ligament forming "groove sign"			

[1]25% of cases of genital ulcers the agent never identified. There is a large overlap in appearance of genital ulcers.

Tick Borne Disease

Lyme Disease

Most common tick borne disease. Usually coast Northeast, Midwest, & West although reported in 43 states. Less than 1/3 recall a tick bite. Bites usually in spring/ summer. <u>Diagnosis</u> – Erythema migrans (EM) is diagnostic if endemic area. Labs are nonspecific with ↑ Sed rate, ↓Hb, normal WBC count (↓lymphocytes) ELISA is positive beyond 2 weeks. IgM peaks 2-6 weeks, and IgG peaks 12 mo into illness (onset ≥ 4 weeks). False ⊕ if syphilis, mono., RMSF, autoimmune disease.	<u>Clinical Stages:</u> *Early local* EM- single lesion ~ 7-10 d after tick bite. Expands centrifugal, clears centrally. Ave 15 cm. See in 75-90% *Early disseminated* (1) many EM lesions 20-50% (2) neuro – lymphocytic meningitis, 7th nerve palsy (↑bilat), radiculoneuritis (3) AV block, myopericarditis (4) ↑spleen, nodes (5) GI – ↑LFTs (6) keratoconjunctivitis, iritis *Late disseminated* – mono-or polyarthritis (esp. large joints), acrodermatitis, retinal vasculitis/optic atrophy, fatigue, dementia, multiple sclerosis-like syndrome.

CDC Criteria for Diagnosis	Treatment
<u>Endemic area</u> [within 2 counties with one definite case or with tick vector] (1) Erythema migrans (EM) with exposure ≤ 30 days from onset OR (2) Laboratory confirmation and > one organ system involved [cardiac, neurologic, arthritis] <u>Nonendemic area</u> (1) EM and > 2 organ systems (2) EM and lab confirmation.	*Early Lyme or mild cardiac disease*– (1) Doxycycline 100 mg PO bid X 10-21 d or (2) Amoxil 250-500 mg PO tid X 10-21 d or (3) cefuroxime 500 mg PO bid X 10-21 d or (4) erythromycin 250 mg PO qid X 10-21 d *Isolated 7th nerve* – above drugs X 30 days *Meningitis, severe cardiac or arthritis* – ceftriaxone 2 g IV qd X 14-21 d or penicillin G 20 million U qd in divided doses X 10-21d
	Clin Infect Dis 2000; 31: 533.

Rocky Mountain Spotted Fever

	Clinical Features	
Most common sites South/South Atlantic (OK, NC #1/#2). Typical rash onset 2-3 days after illness, 1st 1-4 mm macules, later petechiae. Starts ankles/wrists then trunks, palms soles. Complications: encephalitis, pulmonary edema, arrhythmia, GI bleed, skin necrosis, DIC, & neuro deficits. Death in 8-15 days (≤ 5 days if G6PD deficiency) due to hemolysis Labs: Normal WBC, ↓ (platelets, Na, Hb), ↑ (AST, bilirubin, CK, CSF WBC [monocytes] while serological tests are often negative until convalescence.	Fever (88-90% > 102)	88-100%
	Headache/myalgias (each)	83-93%
	Rash anywhere	74-90%
	Rash palms/soles	49-82%
	Tick bite	54-66%
	Triad (fever, headache, rash)	45-67%
	Nausea, vomiting	56-60%
	Other (cough, ↑liver/spleen, abd pain, diarrhea, anorexia, nodes, edema, ataxia, meningismus, stupor, conjunctivitis)	each present in > 10% of patients

Diagnosis	Treatment
(1) Treat based on clinical criteria (e.g. fever, headache, myalgias, with or without rash during summer in endemic areas (2) if rash, direct immunofluoresce stain of skin. (3) Anti-bodies [immune fluorescent antibody] are detected at 7-10 days [altered by treatment] (4) PCR ↓sensitivity (5) Weil-Felix should not be used	(1) doxycycline 100 mg PO or IV bid X 7 days or at least until afebrile for 2 days. (2) chloramphenicol – 500 mg PO or IV qid X 7 days or until afebrile for 2 days. (3) fluoroquinolones may have utility.
	Clin Infect Dis 1998; 27: 1353.

Procedure for Tick Removal

- Apply gloves.
- Consider injecting small wheal of lidocaine + epinephrine directly beneath tick.
- Application of petroleum jelly, isopropyl alcohol, fingernail polish or a hot match to the underside of the tick may actually cause regurgitation (of spirochete & other organisms) and **should be avoided**.
- Using blunt tweezers, grasp the tick as close as possible to the skin.
- Pull slowly in a firm perpendicular direction away from the skin.
- Do not squeeze the tick and do not rotate as pulling away from skin.
- Cleanse area thoroughly after procedure with disinfectant.
- Person performing procedure should thoroughly wash hands afterwards.
- Place tick into alcohol or flush down toilet.

Toxic Shock Syndrome

Toxic shock syndrome is due to toxin (TSST-1) produced by *S. aureus*. TSST-1 sources include tampons (50% of cases), nasal packing, wounds, post partum vaginal colonization and many other sites.

Criteria for Diagnosis - Must have each (•) of following

- Temperature > 38.9 C (102F)
- Systolic BP < 90, orthostatic decrease of Systolic BP 15 mm Hg **or** syncope.
- Rash - diffuse, macular erythroderma, with subsequent desquamation.
- Involvement of *3 of the following* organ systems either clinically **or** by labs.

GI - vomiting, or profuse diarrhea	Muscular - myalgias or ↑ CPK X 2
Renal - ↑ BUN + Cr X 2, sterile pyuria	Heme - platelets < 100,000/mm3
Liver – AST, ALT ↑ X 2	Mucosa - vaginal, conjunctiva, or
CNS - disoriented, nonfocal exam	pharyngeal hyperemia

- Negative serology for Rocky Mountain spotted fever, leptospirosis, measles, hepatitis B, antinuclear antibody, VDRL, monospot; blood, urine, throat cultures.

Management

- Restore intravascular volume with NS. Pressors may be needed. Admit to ICU.
- Obtain blood for CBC, platelets, coagulation studies, electrolytes, liver function tests, culture urine, blood ± CSF. Obtain CXR, arterial blood gas, and ECG.
- Search for focus of infection and remove source (e.g. tampon).
- If bleeding, treat coagulopathy with platelets, fresh frozen plasma or transfuse. Nafcillin or oxacillin 1-2 g IV q 4 h until clinically improved then oral anti-staphy-lococcal agents (dicloxacillin, or 1st generation cephalosporin) for 10-14 days. Consider vancomycin if suspect methicillin resistant *S. aureus*. Note: antibiotics only reduce recurrence of toxic shock and do not treat actual disease.

Kidney/Renal Disorders

Studies useful in Determining Etiology of Acute Renal Failure

Test	Pre-renal	Renal	Post-renal
Urine sodium (mEq/L)	< 20	> 40	> 40
Fractional excretion of sodium[1]	< 1%	> 2%	> 2%
Renal failure index (RFI) [2]	< 1	> 2	> 2
Urine osmolality (mOsm/L)	> 500	< 300	< 400
Urine/serum creatinine ratio	> 40	< 20	< 20
Serum BUN/creatinine ratio	> 20	< 10-20	< 10-20
Renal size by ultrasound	normal	normal	normal or↑
Radionuclide renal scan	↓ uptake ↓ excretion	uptake OK uptake OK	uptake OK ↓ excretion

[1] - FE_{Na} = 100 x (urine Na^+/plasma Na^+) / (urine creatinine/plasma creatinine)

Normal FE_{Na} is 1-2% , [2] - RFI = (urine Na^+) / (urine creatinine / serum creatinine)

Calculation of Creatinine Clearance (CLcr)	• Male CLcr = $\dfrac{[140 - age\ (years)] \times weight\ (kg)}{serum\ creatinine\ (mg/dl) \times 72}$ • For women, multiply above result by 0.85. • Normal creatinine clearance is ~ 100 ml/min

Evaluation of Hematuria

History/exam does not point to specific diagnosis
(e.g. nephrolithiasis, infection, prior failure)

↓

Evaluate urine for (1) RBC morphology (2)
character of sediment & (3) proteinuria

↙ ↘

Medical Disorder/Renal
• Dysmorphic RBCs
• RBC casts
• Proteinuria ≥ 2+

Urologic Disorder
• Normal RBC
• No casts
• Proteinuria ≤ 2+

Renal function tests, US,
biopsy?, Nephrologist

US, IVP, CT (if ? stone),
Cystoscopy, Urologist

Localization Of Hematuria which part of urinary stream?	Total stream	Initial stream	Terminal stream
	Above neck bladder	Anterior urethra	Posterior urethra
	Bladder (stone?)	Urethritis	Bladder neck
	Ureter (tumor?)	Urethral stricture	Bladder trigone
	Kidney (nephritis?)	Meatal stenosis	

Diagnostic Tests

High Yield Criteria for Non-trauma Cranial CT in ED Patients

Clinical Feature	Utility (95% Confidence Intervals)[1]	
• Age 60 years or greater	Sensitivity	100% (94-100)
• Headache with vomiting	Specificity	31% (28-33)
• Focal neurologic deficit	Positive predictive value	11% (8-13)
• Altered mental status	Negative predictive value	100% (98-100)

[1] Utility if one or more feature present   *Acad Emerg Med 1997; 3: 654.*

Dizziness & Vertigo

Dizziness is a vague symptom that manifests as (1) a definite rotational sensation (2) a sensation of impending faint or loss of consciousness (3) dysequilibrium or (4) an ill defined lightheadedness other than vertigo, syncope, or dysequilibrium

Most Common Final Cause of "Dizziness" in ED Patients[1]			
Peripheral vestibular disorder	43%	Hyperventilation	6%
Cardiovascular including vaso-vagal, HTN, CNS disease	21%	Endocrine	5%
		Infectious	4%
Medication	10%	Seizure or Anemia (each 2%)	2%
Post-traumatic	7%	Menière's syndrome	1%
Other	6%	Multiple sensory deficit	1%
Psychogenic	6%	Unknown	10%

Age > 69, focal neuro exam, & absent vertigo identified 86% of patients with a serious cause for "dizziness".   *Ann Emerg Med 1989; 18: 664.*

Vertigo – the illusion of motion

Differentiation of Central (brain stem/cerebellar) from Peripheral Vertigo	
Central Vertigo	*Peripheral Vertigo*
Gradual onset, less intense	Acute onset, intense spinning, swaying
Mild peripheral symptoms	Nausea, vomiting, diaphoresis
Nonfatigable, multidirection nystagmus	Aggravated by change in position
Nystagmus uninhibited by eye fixation	Fatigable, unidirectional nystagmus
Vertical Nystagmus (always central)	Nystagmus inhibited by fixing on object
Focal cerebellar or brain stem findings	Otic symptoms (pain, tinnitus, ↓ hearing).
	No central focal examination findings.

Nylen Barany (Hallpike-Dix) Maneuver

Maneuver – With patient in sitting position and the physician supporting the head, the patient rapidly assumes the supine position with head hanging 45 degrees off bed, 1st with head straight, then head turned 45 degrees to left, then 45 degrees to right.

Peripheral vertigo – The above maneuver elicits vertigo and nystagmus with a latency of several seconds and duration of < 1 minute. Nystagmus is unidirectional and nystagmus/vertigo are fatigable.

Central Vertigo – The above maneuver may elicit nystagmus with no latency, nonfatigable, multidirectional & generally lasts > 1 minute.

Emerg Med Clin North Am 1998; 16: 845.

Benign Paroxysmal Positional Vertigo (BPPV) Repositioning Maneuvers

BPPV is one of most common causes of vertigo and "dizziness" in ED patients (esp. > 50 years old). Free floating debris within the semicircular canals are felt to be responsible for symptoms. The canalith-repositioning procedures outlined below have been found effective for relieving symptoms of BPPV of the posterior semicircular canal & may not be effective if horizontal canal involvement.

Maneuver	Description
Eply Maneuver	• Seat patient & have patient turn head 45 degrees toward **affected** ear (*holding physician's arm for support*) • Lower patient to supine position with head still at 45 degrees toward the affected ear and head hanging off the end of the bed • Hold the patient in this position until nystagmus/vertigo abate (*some recommend holding position for 4 minutes*) • Then, turn head 90 degrees toward alternate ear. • With head still turned, roll the patient onto the side of the unaffected ear (patient is now looking at the floor) • This may precipitate more nystagmus/vertigo (maintain X 3-4 minutes) • Return patient to seated position • Tilt head 30 degrees down toward chest (maintain X 3-4 minutes) • Remain upright, avoid bending over, or driving for 1-2 days
Semont Maneuver	• Seat patient and turn head 45 degrees toward **unaffected** ear • Lower patient – lie affected side/shoulder on gurney (nose up) • Hold position for 3 minutes • Without changing head rotation, quickly move to seated position and then lie opposite shoulder on gurney (nose is now down) X 3 min • Slowly move to seated position • Remain upright, avoid bending over, or driving for 1-2 days

Ann Emerg Med 2001; 37: 392.

Probability of Falling in Patients ≥ 75 years Old

Specific Risk Factor	Total Number of Risk Factors	Probability of Falling per Year
Sedative use		
Cognitive impairment	No risk factors	8%
Lower extremity disability	1 risk factor	19%
Palmomental reflex	2 risk factors	32%
Abnormal balance/gait	3 risk factors	60%
Foot problems	≥4 risk factors	78%

N Engl J Med 1988; 1701.

Get Up & Go Test for Geriatric Mobility

Test: Get up out of a standard armchair, walk 3 m (10 ft), turn, walk back to chair and sit down. Ambulate with or without assistive device & follow above 3 step command. One practice trial & three actual trials are performed with three trials averaged.

	Seconds	Rating
Get Up and Go Predictive Results	< 10	Freely mobile
	10 - 19	Mostly independent
	20 – 29	Variable mobility
	≥ 30	Impaired mobility

Am Fam Physician 2000; 61: 2159.

Headache – see page 109-111 for Subarachnoid & Stroke

Most Frequent Cause of Headaches in 485 Adult ED Patients

Medical Illness	33%	Subarachnoid hemorrhage[1]	0.8%
Muscle contraction – tension	32%	Meningitis	0.8%
Migraine	22%	Neuritis	0.6%
Unidentified	7%	Temporal arteritis	0.4%
CNS tumor	3%	Subdural hematoma	0.2%

[1] Subarachnoid bleed is present in up to 17% of ED patients with worst headache ever.
Ann Emerg Med 1980; 9: 404; Acad Emerg Med 1998; 32: 297.

Weakness

Acute Weakness (Upper vs. Lower Motor Neuron)

Upper motor neuron (UMN) lesions cause damage to cortex (e.g. stroke), brain stem, or spinal cord. Lower motor neuron (LMN) lesions damage the anterior horn cells, the neuromuscular junction or muscle (e.g. muscular dystrophies).

	Category	UMN disease	LMN disease
Differentiation of	Muscular deficit	Muscle groups	Individual muscles
upper motor neuron	Reflexes	↑ (± acutely ↓)	Decreased/absent
from lower motor	Tone	↑ (± acutely ↓)	Decreased
neuron disease	Fasciculations	Absent	Present
	Atrophy	Absent/minimal	Present

Assessment of Acute Muscle Weakness

Assess ventilation: FVC should be $\geq$ 15ml/kg and max. inspiratory force > 15cmH$_2$0

Spinal Cord	Peripheral Neuropathy	Myoneural Junction	Muscle disease
Lower limbs weak	Generally weak	Cranial nerves	Generally weak
Absent lower DTR[1]	General areflexia	Generally weak	Weak proximally
Sharp sensory level	Stocking/glove	Fasciculations	Muscles tender
Bladder/bowel	Sensory loss	No sensory loss	No sensory loss
(B/B) incontinence	OK B/B	OK B/B	OK B/B
↓ examples[2]	↓ examples[2]	↓ examples[2]	↓ examples[2]
transverse myelitis cord tumor/bleed, abscess or disc herniation	Guillain Barre porphyria, arsenic toxic neuropathy tick paralysis	Myasthenia gravis organophosphates botulism	polymyositis alcohol/endocrin myopathy electrolyte abnl[3]

[1] DTR - deep tendon reflexes, [2] - lists are not comprehensive, [3] - abnormality (K, Na, Ca)

Bell's Palsy

A peripheral 7th cranial nerve palsy. Etiology is usually viral (e.g. herpes), but should consider Lyme disease, middle ear infection/lesion, CNS mass, or vascular disease. If forehead not unilaterally weak, obtain neuroimaging study.

Clinical Features		Management
Unilateral forehead weakness	100%	• Exclude CNS and otic disease
Maximum deficit in 96 h	>95%	• Prednisone 50 mg PO qd X 5 days
Maximum deficit in 48 h	50%	• Administer *Lacrilube* to eye & use eye
↑ tearing	68%	patch at night to prevent corneal
Mastoid pain	61%	abrasion.
Abnormal taste	57%	• ± Acyclovir 400 mg PO 5 times/day for
Hyperacusis	29%	10 days (esp. if onset < 3 days)
↓ tearing	16%	• Follow up with neurologist
Numbness (± 5th cranial nerve)	<50%	

Guillain-Barre

Guillain-Barre is post-infectious autoimmune destruction of peripheral nerves. 85-95% have full recovery (weeks to months after weakness progression stops).

Clinical Features	Diagnosis
• Recent viral illness in 50-67%	• Primarily based on clinical features
• Weakness begins symmetrically in legs and ascends to arms and trunk	• CSF – protein normal or > 400 mg/L
	• CSF –WBC normal or monocytosis
• Weak onset rapid↓ or absent DTRs	• Nerve conductions study (slowing)
• Face involvement in 25-50%	**Management**
• Hypesthesias or paresthesias in 33%	• 16-28% require ventilatory support
• Miller-Fischer variant – weakness begins in face and descends with ophthalmoplegia and ataxia	• Plasmapheresis and/or steroids
	• Watch for embolism (consider SC heparin) and infection

Myasthenia Gravis

An autoimmune disease where antibodies destroy acetylcholine receptor at myoneural junction. Thymus abnormalities (thymoma in 10-25%) are often present.

Clinical Features	
• Ptosis, diplopia, blurring (common) • Dysarthria, dysphagia, jaw muscle weakness, head drooping • Asymmetric weakness	• Either truncal or extremity weakness • Weakness worsens with repetition • Heat worsens & cold improves weakness (cold pack improves ptosis)
Myasthenic crisis	Crisis Management
• Due to worsening disease with weakness, difficulty swallowing and respiratory insufficiency. • Precipitants – infection, antibiotics Aminoglycosides, tetracycline, clindamycin), CNS depressants, β blockers, quinidine, procainamide, lidocaine, metabolic (↑K,↑Mg, ↓K,↓Ca)	• Tension test: edrophonium (*Tensilon*) 1-2 mg IV while on cardiac monitor. If no adverse response, give 8 mg IV. Improvement = myasthenic crisis. Worsening = cholinergic crisis. • Assess ventilation – Forced Vital Capacity should be ≥ 15 ml/kg and Maximum inspiratory force should be > 15 cm H_2O
Cholinergic crisis	
• Overdose of anticholinesterase meds. • Weakness occurs with SLUDGE (salivation, lacrimation, urination, defecation, GI upset, and emesis)	• Look for and treat precipitants. • Admit all patients with either a myasthenic crisis or with a cholinergic crisis.

Stroke, TIA, and Subarachnoid Hemorrhage

	Risk Factors	# factors	90 day stroke risk
Risk of Stroke following a Transient Ischemic Attack	Age > 60 years	0	0%
	Diabetes Mellitus	1	3%
	Duration TIA > 10 min	2	7%
	Weakness with TIA	3	11%
	Speech impairment	4	15%
	occurred with TIA	5	34%

JAMA 2000; 284: 2901.

Subarachnoid Hemorrhage (SAH)

Saccular (berry) aneurysms are most common cause (> AV malformations, mycotic aneurysms, anticoagulation or vasculitis). *Risks*: personal or family history, pre-eclampsia, polycystic kidney disease, atherosclerosis, hypertension, alcohol, cigarettes, aspirin, cocaine. Mean age at rupture is 40-60 years. 56% occur at rest, 25% while working, 10% while sleeping.

Clinical features	
Any headache (H/A)	70%
Warning (sentinel) H/A	55%
Neck pain or stiffness	78%
Altered mental status	53%
3rd cranial nerve deficit	9%
Seizure	3-25%
Focal deficit	19%
No H/A, deficit, or nuchal rigidity	11%

Cooperative Aneurysm Study *Neurology* 1983; 33: 981.

Grade	Hunt and Hess Classification of SAH	Normal CT
I	Asymptomatic, minimal headache (H/A) and mild nuchal rigidity	15%
II	Moderate-severe H/A, nuchal rigidity, cranial nerve deficits only	7%
III	Drowsy, confused or mild focal deficit	4%
IV	Stupor, mild/mod hemiparesis, early decerebrate or vegetative Δ	1%
V	Deep coma, decerebrate rigidity, moribund appearance	0%

SAH Diagnosis	SAH Treatment
• CT abnormal > 95% if onset < 12 h	• ↓systolic BP to ≤ 160 mm Hg or MAP to ≤ 110 mm Hg
• CT abnormal 77% if onset > 12 h	• Nimodipine (*Nimotop*) 60 mg PO q6h to decrease vasospasm
• CSF > 100,000 RBC's/ mm^3 (mean) although any # RBC's can be found	
• Xanthochromia (traumatic spinal taps do not cause acute xanthochromia)	• Fosphenytoin/phenytoin prophylaxis
• ECG – peaked, deep or inverted T waves, ↑ QT, or large U waves	• Neurosurgical consult
	• Early angiography & surgical intervention per neurosurgeon

Stroke

Ischemic strokes (85%) are (1) thrombotic (2) embolic or (3) hypoperfusion. Hemorrhagic strokes (15%) are intracerebral or subarachnoid (see below).

Major stroke syndromes

- *Anterior cerebral artery*: paralysis of contralateral leg > arm. Sensory deficits parallel weakness, with altered mentation, gait apraxia, and incontinence.
- *Middle cerebral artery*: paralysis contralateral arm, face > leg. Sensory deficits parallel paralysis, blind (½ visual field), dysphasia, & agnosia.
- *Posterior cerebral artery* (occipital, parietal lobes): Blind in half of visual field, 3rd nerve paralysis, visual agnosia, altered mental status and cortical blindness.
- *Vertebrobasilar artery*: vertigo, nystagmus, dysphagia, facial numbness, dysarthria, contralateral loss of pain, temperature, diplopia, syncope.

Management: See page 110-113

American Heart Association Recommended Studies in Suspected Acute Ischemic Stroke

All patients		If clinically suspected alternate disease	
CT (or MRI)	Renal function	Liver function	Oxygen saturation
EKG	CBC/platelets	Toxicology screen	CXR
Glucose	PT/INR	Blood alcohol	Lumbar puncture
Electrolytes	PTT	Pregnancy test	EEG

American Heart Association (AHA) Suspected Stroke Algorithm

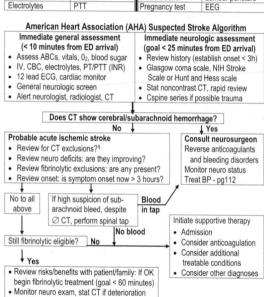

Immediate general assessment (< 10 minutes from ED arrival)
- Assess ABCs, vitals, O₂, blood sugar
- IV, CBC, electrolytes, PT/PTT (INR)
- 12 lead ECG, cardiac monitor
- General neurologic screen
- Alert neurologist, radiologist, CT

Immediate neurologic assessment (goal < 25 minutes from ED arrival)
- Review history (establish onset < 3h)
- Glasgow coma scale, NIH Stroke Scale or Hunt and Hess scale
- Stat noncontrast CT, rapid review
- Cspine series if possible trauma

Does CT show cerebral/subarachnoid hemorrhage?

No → **Probable acute ischemic stroke**
- Review for CT exclusions?[1]
- Review neuro deficits: are they improving?
- Review fibrinolytic exclusions: are any present?
- Review onset: is symptom onset now > 3 hours?

Yes → **Consult neurosurgeon**
Reverse anticoagulants and bleeding disorders
Monitor neuro status
Treat BP - pg112

No to all above

If high suspicion of sub-arachnoid bleed, despite ∅ CT, perform spinal tap

Blood in tap →

No blood ↓

Initiate supportive therapy
- Admission
- Consider anticoagulation
- Consider additional treatable conditions
- Consider other diagnoses

Still fibrinolytic eligible? | **No** →

↓ **Yes**

- Review risks/benefits with patient/family: If OK begin fibrinolytic treatment (goal < 60 minutes)
- Monitor neuro exam, stat CT if deterioration
- Admit to critical care unit
- No anticoagulants or antiplatelet Rx for 24 h

[1] - edema, sulcal effacement, mass effect or possible hemorrhage

AHA/ACC. _Circulation_ 2000; 102 (suppl I): I-204-I-216.

Thrombolytic (rTPA) use in Acute Ischemic Stroke

Indications for rTPA[1] use in Acute Ischemic Stroke[2, 3]	Age 18-80 years
	Onset of symptoms ≤ 3 hours before treatment initiated
	No CT evidence of bleeding or major early infarct (below)
	Acute focal neurologic deficits excluding contraindications

[1] rTPA - tissue plasminogen activator. (Streptokinase is NOT used for acute stroke)
[2] Facilities administering rTPA should have ability to manage intracranial bleeding.
[3] Some published studies on fibrinolytic therapy in stroke treated at community hospitals show worse outcome than traditional therapy. Fibrinolytic therapy for stroke should be performed in the context of a well established hospital protocol.

JAMA 2000; 283: 1151 Neurology 1996; 47: 835. Stroke 2003; 34: 1056, 1106.
(www.strokeaha.org)

Contraindications to rTPA Use in Acute Ischemic Stroke

Any known or suspected CNS bleed (current or prior history)	Active bleed or acute trauma (e.g. fracture)
Recent CNS surgery, trauma, or stroke[2]	CT with major early infarct signs[1]
Subarachnoid bleed suspected	Use caution if NIH stroke scale > 20-22[4]
Noncompressible arterial puncture in past 7 days	Use caution if mild or rapidly improving deficit (e.g. NIH stroke scale ≤ 5)
Myocardial infarction in past 3 months	Pregnancy or lactating females
Recent spinal tap	*Known bleeding diathesis including:*
Blood glucose < 50 or > 400 mg/dl	• warfarin use or PT > 15 (INR >1.5)
Uncontrolled HTN[3] (BP ≥ 185/110)	• Platelets < 100,000/mm³
Seizure at onset of stroke	• heparin use ≤ 48 hours or high PTT
GI or GU bleeding in prior 21 days	*Isolated mild neurologic deficit below*
Non-CNS major surgery in prior 14 days	• ataxia • dysarthria
CNS neoplasm, or aneurysm	• sensory loss • mild weakness

[1] - edema, sulcal effacement, mass effect or possible hemorrhage. [2] - prior 3 months
[3] HTN - hypertension (after treatment), [4] See page 113 for NIH stroke scale.
Neurology 1996; 47: 835. Stroke 2003; 34: 1056. (www.strokeaha.org)

Protocol for rTPA Administration

- Administer rtPA 0.9 mg/kg (max dose of 90 mg) with 10% given as IV bolus followed by infusion of remaining drug over 60 minutes.
- Monitor arterial blood pressure during ensuing 24 hours
  (1) Monitor q 15 min X 1st 2 hours   (3) Then q 60 min for next 16 hours
  (2) Then q 30 min for next 6 hours   (4) Treat blood pressure (see below)
- Do not administer aspirin, heparin, warfarin, ticlopidine or other antiplatelet or antithrombotic agents within 24 hours of rtPA treatment.
- Do not place central venous line or perform arterial punctures in first 24 hours.
- Do not place bladder catheter for 30 min or NG tube for 24 hours after infusion.

Management of Blood Pressure in Acute Ischemic Stroke

Not Eligible for Thrombolytics	
Blood Pressure[1]	**Management**
Systolic BP < 220 OR Diastolic BP < 120	• Only treat if end organ damage (e.g. aortic dissection, MI, pulmonary edema, hypertensive encephalopathy). • Treat symptoms (e.g. headache, nausea, vomiting, pain or agitation) as needed. • Treat acute complications (e.g. hypoxia, ↑ICP, seizures, or hypoglycemia) if needed.
Systolic BP > 220 OR Diastolic BP < 121-140	• Labetalol 10-20 mg IV over 1-2 minutes, may repeat or double q 10 minutes to maximum total dose 300 mg OR • Nicardipine 5 mg/hour IV infusion initially, titrate to desired effect by increasing 2.5 mg/hour q 5 minutes to maximum of 15 mg/hour • GOAL: 10-15% reduction of blood pressure
Diastolic BP > 140	• Nitroprusside 0.5 micrograms/kg/min IV as initial dose with continuous BP monitoring • GOAL: 10-15% reduction of blood pressure
Eligible for Thrombolytic Therapy - Pretreatment	
Systolic BP > 185 OR Diastolic BP > 110	• Labetalol 10-20 mg IV over 1-2 minutes, may repeat X 1 OR Nitropaste 1-2 inches • If BP is not reduced and maintained with SBP < 185 AND Diastolic BP < 110 do not give thrombolytics
Thrombolytic Therapy - Posttreatment	
Check BP q 15 min X 2 hours, then q 30 min X 6 hours, then q hour X 16 hours	
Diastolic BP > 140	• Nitroprusside 0.5 microgram/kg/min as initial dose and titrate to desired blood pressure
Systolic BP > 230 OR Diastolic BP > 121-140	• Labetalol 10 mg IV over 1-2 minutes, may repeat or double q 10 minutes to maximum total dose 300 mg OR give initial bolus and then start drip at 2-8 mg/min OR • Nicardipine 5 mg/hour IV infusion initially, titrate to desired effect by increasing 2.5 mg/hour q 5 minutes to maximum of 15 mg/hour. • If BP not controlled by above consider nitroprusside
Systolic BP 180-230 OR Diastolic BP 105-120	• Labetalol 10 mg IV over 1-2 minutes, may repeat or double q 10 minutes to maximum total dose 300 mg OR give initial bolus and then start drip at 2-8 mg/min

BP – blood pressure in mm Hg   *Stroke* 2003; 34: 1056. (www.strokeaha.org)

National Institute of Health Stroke Scale

1a. Level of consciousness (LOC)	Alert	0	**6. Best motor leg** [2] No drift in 5 sec.	0
	Arouses to obey respond, answers	1	Drift without hitting bed/support– 5 sec.	1
	Responds to pain	2	Drifts completely down in 5 sec.	2
	Autonomic reflexes or no response	3	No effort - limb falls immediately	3
			No movement	4
1b. LOC questions *(ask age & current month)*	Both correct	0	*(6a. left leg, 6b. right leg)*	
	One correct	1	**7. Limb ataxia** [3] Absent	0
	Incorrect	2	Present in one limb	1
1c. LOC commands *(make fist, close eyes)*	Obeys both	0	Present in two limbs	2
	Obeys one	1	*Absent (0) if can't understand or paralysis*	
	Incorrect	2	**8. Sensory** Normal	0
2. Best gaze	Normal	0	Partial loss– less sharp pinprick	1
	Partial	1	Not aware of being touched	2
Forced deviation or total gaze paresis not overcome by oculocephalic reflex		2	**9. Best language** [4] No aphasia	0
3. Best visual	No loss	0	*Mild/moderate aphasia* – loss of fluency or comprehension. Can identify material or content of pictures	1
	Partial hemianopsia	1	*Severe aphasia* – fragmented expression Cant ID material from patient response	2
	Complete hemianopsia	2	Mute, aphasia – no comprehension	3
	Bilateral hemianopsia	3	**10. Dysarthria** [5] Normal	0
4. Facial palsy	None	0	Mild-moderate – understand slurring	1
	Minor asymmetry with smile	1	Severe – unintelligible	2
	Partial (near total paralysis low face)	2	**11.Extinction/Inattention (Neglect)** None	0
	Complete	3	Visual, tactile, auditory, spatial, personal inattention or extinction to bilateral stimulation in one of senses tested	1
5. Best motor arm [1]	No drift in 10 sec.	0		
	Drift without hitting bed/support– 10 sec.	1		
	Drifts completely down in 10 sec.	2	Profound hemi-inattention or extinction to > 1 mode (does not recognize hand or orients to only one side of space)	2
	No effort - limb falls immediately	3		
	No movement	4		
www.ninds.nih.gov/doctorsNIH Stroke Scale (version 10-03).				

1 Arm drift – 1 arm pronates from 90 degree or 45 degree elevation (10 second test)
2 Leg drift - While supine, 1 leg falls to bed from 30 degree elevation (5 second test)
3 Test finger-nose, heel to shin both sides. Ataxia only if out of proportion to weakness.
4 Aphasia – disturbance in processing language. Patient often uses inappropriate words or nonfluent sentences. Test *receptive aphasia* by having patient follow simple commands and test *expressive aphasia* by identifying objects.
5 Dysarthria – slurring from paralysis or incoordination of muscles for speech

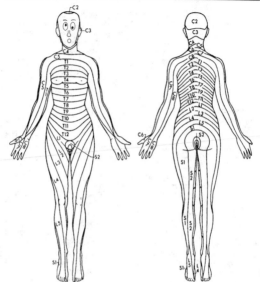

Motor level	Motor function
C1-2	neck flexion
C3	side neck flexion
C4	spontaneous breathing
C5	shoulder abduction/deltoid
C6	biceps (elbow flexion), wrist extension
C7	triceps, wrist flexion
C8	thumb ext, ulnar deviation
C8/T1	finger flexion
T1-T12	intercostal and abdominal muscles

Motor level	Motor function
T7-L1	abdominal muscles
T12	cremasteric reflex
L1/L2	hip flexion, psoas
L2/3/4	hip adduction, quads
L4	foot dorsiflexion, foot inversion
L5	great toe dorsiflexion
S1	foot plantar flexion, foot eversion
S2-S4	rectal tone

Diagnosis of Ectopic Pregnancy in Clinically Stable Patients

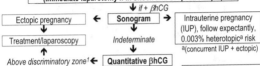

Qualitative βhCG or immediate bedside ultrasound if available
(Immediate laparotomy if in shock and suspect ectopic)

⬇ *if + βhCG*

Ectopic pregnancy ← **Sonogram** → Intrauterine pregnancy (IUP), follow expectantly, 0.003% heterotopic[a] risk

[a](concurrent IUP + ectopic)

Treatment/laparoscopy

⬆
Above discriminatory zone[1] ← **Quantitative βhCG**

Below discriminatory zone (DZ)[1]

1. progesterone levels < 5 ng/ml are ~ 95% predictive of abnormal pregnancy.
2. progesterone levels > 25 ng/ml indicate a 97% chance that pregnancy is normal
3. no single cutoff is 100% accurate

Options
1. serial βhCG →
2. laparoscopy
3. progesterone
4. culdocentesis

Brennan *Acad Emerg Med* 1995; 1081

Repeat βhCG in 48 h
1. if ↓ or →: ectopic or abortion or nonviable pregnancy
2. < 66% ↑βhCG occurs in ectopics, abortions and in 15% of normal pregnancies.
3. > 66%↑βhCG occurs IUP and also in up to 15% of ectopic pregnancies.

[1] DZ is 1000-1,500 mIU/ml for transvaginal US & 6,500 mIU/ml for transabdominal US

Ultrasound (US) Findings[1]
Intrauterine pregnancy (IUP)
1. Decidual reaction
2. Gestational sac seen at 4.5 wk with βhCG > 1000-1400 via transvaginal US or 6 wk with βhCG > 6,500 via transabdominal US
3. Yolk sac - see at 5.5 weeks (βhCG > 7200)
4. Fetal pole/heart beat are seen at 5.5 to to 7 weeks (βhCG > 10,800-17,200)
Ectopic pregnancy (% with finding)
1. Empty uterus, decidual reaction, or pseudosac (10-20%)
2. Cul-de-sac fluid (24-63%):echogenic=blood
3. Adnexal mass (60-90%)
4. Echogenic halo around tube (26-68%)
5. Fetal heart activity (8-23%)

Quantitative βhCG in IUP [2,3]

Time	mIU/ml
< 1 week	< 5 - 50
1 - 2 weeks	40 - 300
2 - 3 weeks	100 - 1,000
3 - 4 weeks	500 - 6,000
1 - 2 months	5,000 - 200,000
2 - 3 months	10,000 - 100,000
2nd trimester	3,000 - 50,000
3rd trimester	1,000 - 50,000

[1] Transvaginal sonography unless otherwise stated
[2] Time from conception
[3] Median time for βhCG to turn negative after spontaneous abortion is 16 days (30 days for elective)

Difficult Deliveries (Breech and Shoulder Dystocia)

Techniques described are for instances when obstetrical expertise is unavailable and ED delivery is required. Call for OB back-up immediately for these occasions.

Breech Delivery	Mariceau maneuver
• Grasp both feet index finger between ankles & pull feet through vulva. Wrap feet in towel, perform episiotomy	• Next, extract head using Mariceau maneuver. Apply suprapubic pressure, gently flex head by pressing on maxilla

• Apply downward traction until hips delivered, with thumbs over sacrum & fingers over hip, continue down traction.
• As scapula emerges rotate back laterally
• Attempt shoulder delivery only after low scapula & axilla visible.
• 1st deliver anterior shoulder/arm, then rotate and deliver posterior arm
• If unable, deliver posterior shoulder 1st – pull feet up above Mom's groin, ± guide 2 fingers along humerus + gently sweep fetal arm down. Arm may be delivered by depression of body alone or with finger sweep as per posterior shoulder.
• Rotate occiput anteriorly as in diagram.

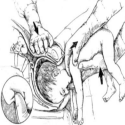

Used with permission. Williams Obstetrics. Appleton & Lange 1997; 501 (Figure 21-11)

Maneuvers for Managing Shoulder Dystocia

• 1st McRoberts maneuver (hyperflex hips–rotates hips cephalad & flattens lumbar lordosis) + assistant applies suprapubic pressure. Assistant's pressure may be applied as an anterior to posterior (Mazzanti) or lateral to medial maneuver. (79% success)
• Gaskin maneuver – hand/knee position –allows post. shoulder descent (83% success)
• Wood's screw (**below**) – push posterior shoulder anteriorly 180° & deliver this shoulder
• Rubin – push (adduct) either shoulder to ant. fetal chest 15-30° (↓ bisacromial diameter)
• Clavicle fracture – pull upward, anteriorly on distal clavicle to ↓ bisacromial diameter.

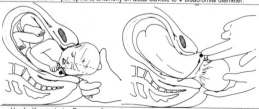

Used with permission Romney. Gynecology and Obstetrics: The Health Care of Women . Figure 75-14, New York. McGraw-Hill Book Co, 1975.

Pregnancy Induced Hypertension - Preeclampsia - Eclampsia

Pregnancy induced hypertension (PIH)	
• BP ≥ 140/90 mm Hg **Or** • BP ↑of ≥ 30/15 above prior BP	Measure BP on 2 occasions ≥ 6 hours apart (not practical in the ED)

Pre-eclampsia	Severe pre-eclampsia
• Hypertension with general edema or proteinuria > 20 weeks gestation • Weight gain > 2 lb./week or 6lbs/month is suggestive • Proteinuria occurs late: > 300 mg protein/24h (300 mg/d = 1+ dipstick) or > 1 g/L on 2 urines > 6h apart	• BP ≥ 160/110 mm Hg • Proteinuria ≥ 2+, Cr > 1.2 mg/dl-new • Oliguria (urine output ≤ 500 ml/24h) • Elevated AST/ALT • Platelets < 100,000 cells/μL • Headache, visual Δ, abdominal pain, pulmonary edema, hyperreflexia

HELLP syndrome	ECLAMPSIA
• Hemolytic anemia, Elevated Liver function tests, Low Platelets • Variant of pre-eclampsia with upper abdominal pain and/or vomiting • Minimal hypertension	• Seizures due to pre-eclampsia in 3rd trimester or ≤ 7 d of delivery (± later) • This is the most common cause of death in Pregnancy Induced Hypertension (PIH)

Treatment of Pre-eclampsia/Eclampsia

- *Seizure prophylaxis* - <u>Load</u> 4-6 g MgSO₄ IV in 100 ml NS over 30 min. <u>Maintenance</u>: Add 20 g MgSO₄ to 500 ml NS and administer at 50 ml/h (2g/h). Continue through labor and 12 h after delivery. Side effects: flushing, headache, blurring, dizziness, ↓reflexes, respiratory and cardiac arrest.   Monitor patellar reflexes, respirations and keep urine output ≥ 25 ml/h.
  <u>Antidote to MgSO₄ overdose</u>: Calcium gluconate (10%) 10-20 ml slow IV push.
  <u>Contraindications</u> to MgSO₄: myasthenia gravis, maternal cardiovascular disease, renal impairment, or use of nifedipine, β agonists, and steroids as use of these drugs with MgSO₄ may lead to pulmonary edema/cardiac depression.
- *Seizure treatment* - Barbiturates and benzodiazepines (esp short-acting, eg. midazolam) recommended - both may cause fetal depression. (see page 140).
- *Antihypertensives* - Indications - diastolic BP is ≥ 105 mmHg. Goal - ↓diastolic BP to 90-95 mmHg (lower if baseline diastolic BP is known to be < 75 mmHg).
  1. <u>Hydralazine</u> - 5 mg IV over 1-2 min. Repeat 5-10 mg IV q 20-30 min prn. If a total of 20 mg given without effect, try 2ⁿᵈ drug.
  2. <u>Labetalol</u> - 10 mg IV. Double q 10 min until BP goal or max. 300 mg (total).
  3. <u>Diazoxide</u> - Administer 30 mg IV q 5-15 min prn (max dose 150 mg).

Third Trimester Vaginal Bleeding and Post Partum Hemorrhage

Placental Abruption (Separation of Normal Placenta prior to Birth)

Risk factors	Management
• Hypertension, maternal age > 35 y	• Avoid digital pelvic examination until
• Smoking, cocaine use, trauma	placenta previa excluded.
• Causes 30% of 3rd trimester bleeds	• Ultrasound is only 25% sensitive.

Clinical Features		
• Vaginal bleeding (dark)	78%	• Administer O_2, and IV NS.
• Abdominal pain	66%	• Obtain type & crossmatch, PT/PTT,
• Uterine contractions	17%	CBC fibrinogen, platelets, fibrin
• Fetal death	15%	degradation products.
• Maternal DIC[1]	-	• Administer blood, FFP, platelets prn
		• Immediate delivery

[1]bedside DIC screen: place 5 ml maternal venous blood in red top tube, DIC if no clots by 6 min

Placenta Previa

Defined	Management
• Implanted placenta over cervical os	• If pre-term – consider tocolysis with
Clinical Features/Diagnosis	(1) terbutaline 0.25 mg SC q 30 min
• 20-30% of 3rd trimester bleeding	up to 1 mg in 4 hours or
• Sudden profuse vaginal bleeding	(2) terbutaline 2.5-5 mg PO q4-6h or
• Absence of abdominal pain	(3) ritodrine 0.05 mg/kg/min IV,
• Soft non-tender uterus	increase 0.05 mg/min until effect
• **AVOID** digital pelvic examination	(typical range 0.15-0.35 mg/min)
• Ultrasound is 95% sensitive	(4) $MgSO_4$ 4-6 g IV (slow) + 2g/h IV
	• If viable pregnancy (near term) –
	delivery via cesarean section

Postpartum Hemorrhage

Definition	Most common causes
Postpartum hemorrhage is the loss of > 500 ml of blood in 1st 24 h after delivery	• Uterine atony
	• Cervical and uterine lacerations

Management

1. IV NS, blood prn, oxygen, and fundal massage.
2. oxytocin (*Pitocin*) 10 U IM or 10-40 U in 1L NS at 100-200 ml/h after placental delivery - may↓BP **or** methylergonovine tartrate (*Methergine*) 0.2 mg IM after placenta delivers - may cause ↑or↓BP, seizures, headaches
3. 15-methyl $PGF_2\alpha$ (*Carboprost*) 0.25 mg IM q 15-90 min to maximum dose of 2 mg. May↓O_2, so apply pulse oximeter. Use caution if ↑BP, cardiac, hepatic, renal, lung disease, epilepsy, ↓Hb or diabetes.
4. Surgery may be needed for severe bleeding.
5. Consider cervical or uterine laceration, uterine rupture, or abnormal placental attachment if continued bleeding.

Rh Isoimmunization

Kleihauer Betke test estimates blood transfused into maternal circulation. (fetal cells/maternal cells X maternal blood volume [L] = fetomaternal hemorrhage [ml]).

(1) <u>RhIG</u> (Rh Immune globulin/*RhoGAM*) - 1 vial IM is indicated if fetal RBC's possibly entered circulation of Rh negative mother. 1 RhIG vial contains ~ 300 µg of immune globulin and protects against transfusion of 15 ml of Rh⁺ packed RBC's.

(2) <u>RhIG</u> (*MICRhoGAM, MiniGamulin Rh, HypRho-D Mini Dose*) - 1/6 dose neutralizes 2.5 ml RBC's. Indications - pregnancy termination, or ectopic ≤12weeks.[1]

Indications for RhIG therapy

Rh negative mother and one of the following

• Delivery of Rh positive infant	• Threatened abortion (*controversial*) [1]
• Abortion or ectopic pregnancy	• Following amniocentesis, chorionic villi or umbilical blood sampling
• Following trauma (even if minor)	
• Any transfusion of Rh positive blood	• At 28 weeks

[1]Use of Rhogam is controversial in spontaneous or elective abortion < 12 weeks. Some authors recommend its use (Society of Obstetricians and Gynaecologist of Canada, J Obstet Gynaecol Can 2003; 765) while others do not recommend its use (J Reprod Med 2002; 47; 909)

Emerg Med Clin N Am 1994; 12: 257

Dysfunctional Uterine Bleeding - DUB

Exogenous steroids (birth control pills) and anovulatory cycles are most common cause. During evaluation, exclude pregnancy and treatable disorders: infection, trauma, bleeding disorders (20% of hospitalized adolescents with DUB - esp. Von Willebrand's disease), endocrine disorders, tumors, fibroids, and cysts.

Classification, Diagnosis, and Management

Class	Hemoglobin	Management [1]
Mild	> 11 g/dl	(1) Iron supplementation, gynecology follow up
Moderate *NOTE:* *High dose hormone therapy may cause nausea & vomiting*	9-11 g/dl without signs of volume depletion	(1) 4 BCP[2] pills (estrogen/progestin) PO qd until bleeding stops, then taper over 1 week to 1 PO qd **OR** (2) Medroxyprogesterone (*Provera*)[3] 30-40 mg PO qd X 1 week decreasing by 10 mg qd until 10 mg/day, then continue X 3-4 weeks. If bleeding does not stop by 1 week,↑ to 40-50 mg PO qd, then taper. This agent will NOT protect against pregnancy, use other birth control. (3) nonsteroidals (e.g. ibuprofen) lower prostaglandin E₂, + decrease bleeding + Iron and gynecology follow-up
Severe	< 9 or hypo-volemia (e.g.↓BP or ↑heart rate)	(1) Fluid, blood, and dilation & curettage as needed (2) Premarin 25 mg IV or PO q 6-12 h until bleeding stops. (max 4 doses). Then start norethindrone 5 mg PO bid alone or in combination with oral estrogen monophasic BCP (see below) X 4 weeks.

[1] Use caution with administration of listed agents if ≥ 35 or cardiopulmonary disease, as cardiac ischemia, and thromboembolic disease risk is increased with these medicines.

[2] BCP - Birth control pill – estrogen + progestins (e.g.*Lo/Ovral, Ortho-Novum 1/50*)

[3] Alternate regimen - *Provera* 10 mg PO qd, increasing dose 10 mg/day until bleeding stops. Once bleeding controlled, this dose can be maintained for total of 3-4 weeks.

Emerg Med Reports 1996; 219; Obstet Gynecol Clin North Am 2000; 27: 287.

Visual Acuity Screen

96
20/800

873
20/400

2 8 4 3   O X X   20/200

6 3 8 5 2   X O O   20/100

8 7 4 5 9   O X O   20/70

6 3 9 2 5   X O X   20/50

4 2 8 3 6 5   o X o   20/40

3 7 4 2 5 8   x x o   20/30

9 3 7 8 2 6   x o o   20/25

Hold card in good light 14 inches from eye. Record vision for each eye separately with and without glasses. Presbyopic patients should read through bifocal glasses. Myopic patients should wear glasses only.

Pupil Diameter (mm)

. ② ③ ④ ⑤ ⑥ 7 8 9

JG Rosenbaum. Pocket Vision Screen. Beachwood. Ohio

Neuro-Ophthalmology

Anisocoria (Asymmetric pupils) Evaluation - Assuming no CNS trauma

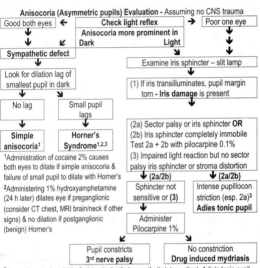

Good both eyes ← **Check light reflex** → Poor one eye

Anisocoria more prominent in

Dark   Light

Sympathetic defect

Look for dilation lag of smallest pupil in dark

No lag   Small pupil lags

Simple anisocoria[1]   **Horner's Syndrome[1,2,3]**

[1]Administration of cocaine 2% causes both eyes to dilate if simple anisocoria & failure of small pupil to dilate with Horner's

[2]Administering 1% hydroxyamphetamine (24 h later) dilates eye if preganglionic (consider CT chest, MRI brain/neck if other signs) & no dilation if postganglionic (benign) Horner's

Examine iris sphincter – slit lamp

(1) If iris transilluminates, pupil margin torn - **Iris damage is present**

(2a) Sector palsy or iris sphincter **OR**
(2b) Iris sphincter completely immobile
Test 2a + 2b with pilocarpine 0.1%
(3) If no sector palsy iris sphincter or stroma distortion

(2a/2b) Sphincter not sensitive or **(3)**

(2a/2b) Intense pupillocon striction (esp. 2a)[3] **Adies tonic pupil**

Administer Pilocarpine 1%

Pupil constricts **3rd nerve palsy**

No constriction **Drug induced mydriasis**

[3] Horner's – ptosis, miosis, facial anhydrosis (sympathetic interruption), Adie's tonic pupil– difficulty in accommodation (esp. young women with reduced DTRs)

Ptosis

To measure levator palpebrae superioris function (1) fix brow position and have patient look down – set lid margin at 0 on a ruler then (2) have patient look up and measure movement of upper lid margin. Normal levator movement is > 12 mm. Ptosis with > 12 mm movement is seen in levator dehiscence and Horner's syndrome, while < 12 mm is seen in myasthenia gravis, 3rd nerve palsy, myopathy (myotonic dystrophy) and congenital ptosis.

Common Causes of Red or Inflamed Eye

Feature	Conjunctivitis	Acute iritis	Acute glaucoma	Cornea trauma or infection
Discharge	moderate-high	none	none	watery,purulent
Vision	normal	sl. blurred	very blurred	usually blurred
Pain	none	moderate	severe	mod/severe
Photophobia	Minimal- none	severe	consensual[1]	Mild-moderate
Conjunctival injection	diffuse, esp. near fornices	mainly circumcorneal	diffuse or perilimbal	diffuse
Pupil	normal	small	mod dilate/fixed	normal
Light response	normal	poor	none	normal
IOP[2]	normal	normal or ↑	elevated	normal
Slit lamp examination	clear anterior chamber	cell and flare reaction	corneal edema, appears steamy	positive fluorescein stain
Gram stain	± organisms	negative	negative	± organisms

[1] pain while shining light in unaffected eye, [2]IOP - Intraocular pressure normally is ≤ 20mmHg.

Conversion Chart for Schiotz Tonometer

Tonometer reading	Tonometer load in grams				Tonometer reading	Tonometer load in grams			
	5.5g	7.5g	10g	15g		5.5g	7.5g	10g	15g
	pressure in mmHg					pressure in mmHg			
0.0	42	59	82	128	7.0	12	18	27	47
0.5	38	54	75	118	7.5	11	17	25	43
1.0	35	50	69	109	8.0	10	16	23	40
1.5	32	46	64	101	8.5	9	14	21	38
2.0	29	42	59	94	9.0	8.5	13	20	35
2.5	27	39	55	88	9.5	8	12	18	32
3.0	24	36	51	81	10.0	7	11	17	30
3.5	22	33	47	76	10.5	7	10	15	27
4.0	21	30	43	71	11	6	9	14	25
4.5	19	28	41	67	12	5	7	12	21
5.0	17	26	37	62	13	4	6	10	20
5.5	16	24	34	58	14	3	5	8	15
6.0	15	22	32	54	15	-	4	6	13
6.5	13	20	29	50	17.5	-	-	4	8

Intraocular pressure (IOP) is falsely ↑ if sticky Schiotz plunger, blinking, accommodation, or looking toward nose. IOP is falsely ↓ with repeated measurements, myopia, anticholinesterase drugs, overhydration and scleral buckle operations.

Acute Narrow Angle Glaucoma

Clinical Features	Treatment
• Headache, vomiting, eye pain • Red eye, perilimbal edema • Conjunctival edema with "flare and cell" in anterior chamber • Mid-dilated, poorly reactive pupil • Intraocular pressure often > 50 mm Hg	• Pilocarpine (2-4%) – 2 drops q 15 min X 2 h or until pupilloconstriction • Pilocarpine 1 drop to unaffected eye • Timolol (*Timoptic*) 0.1% 1 drop • Acetazolamide 500 mg IV, IM or PO • Mannitol 0.5 - 1g/kg IV • Laser or surgical iridectomy

Central Retinal Artery Occlusion

Causes	Clinical Features
• Cardiac, carotid, vascular disease • Hyperviscosity, diabetes, sickle cell,	• Sudden painless unilateral ↓ vision • Afferent pupil defect (no direct reaction to light, + reaction if light shone in contralateral eye) • Narrow retinal arterioles or "boxcars" from segmentation of arteriolar blood • Infarcted retina turns gray • Cherry red macula due to thin retina with clear view of underlying vessels
Treatment	
• Best to start within 2 h (try up to 48h) • Globe pressure/massage on 5 sec and off 5 sec for 5-30 minutes • ↑pCO₂ by breathing in bag or 95%O₂/5%CO₂ mixture • Paracentesis by ophthalmologist	

Treatment cell uses: ↑pCO_2 by breathing in bag or 95%O_2/5%CO_2 mixture

Iritis

<u>Defined</u> – acute inflammation of anterior uvea. <u>Clinical features</u> - ↓ vision, perilimbal redness, photophobia (consensual photophobia) ± ↑ IOP. Slit lamp reveals cell & flare in anterior chamber.	<u>Treatment</u> – (1) IV antibiotics if infection (2) Homatropine 2% or 5% - 1 drop qid (3) Prednisolone 1% - 1 drop qid (4) Systemic nonsteroidal agents (4) Consult ophthalmologist

Temporal Arteritis

History		Examination	
• Mean age (years)	70	• ↓Temp. artery (TA) pulse	46%
• Polymyalgia rheumatica	39%	• Tender temporal artery (TA)	27%
• Headache	68%	• Indurated, red (TA)	23%
• Jaw claudication	45%	• Large artery bruit	21%
• Unilateral vision loss	14%	• Afferent pupil, cranial nerve	-
• Claudication, eye pain, fever	<5%	palsies, pale, swollen disc	-

Diagnosis	Management
• ESR > 50 mm in most cases • Artery biopsy (not emergent)	• Prednisone 60-80 mg PO q day • Ophthalmology consult

Mydriatics/Cycloplegics

Drug *Trade Name*	Duration	Effect[1]	Indication	Comments
Atropine 0.5-3.0%	2 weeks	M, C	dilation	caution if narrow glaucoma
Cyclopentolate HCl *Cyclogyl* 0.5-2%	24 hours	M, C	dilation e.g. exam	same as atropine
Homatropine 2-5%	10-48hours	M, C	dilation	same as atropine
Phenylephrine HCl *Neosynephrine* 0.12-10%	2-3 hours	M	dilation, no cycloplegia	caution: cardiac disease, glaucoma or hypertension
Scopolamine HBr *Hyoscine* 0.25%	2-7 days	M, C	strong cycloplegia	same caution above with dizziness, disorientation
Tropicamide *Mydriacyl* 0.5-1%	6 hours	M, C	dilation, cycloplegia	same as atropine, only weak cycloplegia

[1] M - mydriatic (pupillodilation), C - cycloplegia. Usual dose of meds listed is 1 drop qd – tid. Higher doses may be used for specific diseases (e.g. acute angle glaucoma pg 122).

Note: Traumatic orthopedic injuries including cervical, thoracic, lumbosacral, pelvic, knee, ankle, shoulder and spinal cord injuries are described in the Trauma section of the text (pages 175, 176)

Arthritis and Joint Fluid Analysis

Analysis of Joint Fluid

	Normal	Noninflammatory	Inflammatory	Septic
Clarity	Clear	Clear	Cloudy	Purulent/turbid
Color	Clear	Yellow or blood	Yellow	Yellow
WBC/ml	< 200	<200-2000	200-50,000	> 5000-50000
PMN (%)	< 25%	< 25%	> 75%	> 75%
Crystals	Absent	Absent	May be present	Absent
Glucose[1]	95-100%	95-100%	80-100%	< 50%
Culture	Negative	Negative	Negative	Positive > 50%
Disease	–	Osteoarthritis, trauma, rheumatic fever	Gout, pseudogout, spondyloarthropathy RA[2], Lyme, lupus	Nongonococcal and gonococcal septic arthritis

1 Ratio of joint fluid to serum glucose X 100%, 2 rheumatoid arthritis

Etiology of Arthritis Based on Number of Involved Joints

Monoarthritis (1 joint)	Trauma, Tumor Infection (septic arthritis) Gout or Pseudogout	Lyme disease Avascular necrosis Osteoarthritis (acutely)
Oligoarthritis (2-3 joints)	Lyme disease Rheumatic fever Reiter's syndrome	Gonococcal arthritis Ankylosing spondilitis Polyarticular gout
Polyarthritis (> 3 joints)	Rheumatoid arthritis Lupus	Viral (Rubella, hepatitis) Osteoarthritis (acute)

Etiology of Migratory Arthritis

Gonococcal arthritis, viral arthritis, Rheumatic fever, Lyme disease Subacute bacterial endocarditis Pulmonary infection Mycoplasma, histoplasmosis, coccidioidomycosis	Systemic lupus erythematous Drug hypersensitivity (esp. cefaclor) Septicemia (staphylococcus, streptococcus, meningococcus, & *Neisseria gonorrhea*) Henoch-Schonlein purpura

Brachial Plexus Injuries

Etiology- trauma, infection, hematoma, vascular occlusion or cancer.
Sensory loss – generally incomplete/inconsistent

Injury	Muscles *(sites of weakness)*	Reflex lost
Upper trunk[1]	Supra-infraspinatus (shoulder rotation), bicep, deltoid, pronator teres, brachioradialis	Biceps
Middle trunk	Latissimus, triceps, extensor digitorum comm (finger extension), ext. carpi radialis (wrist extension)	Triceps
Low trunk *Klumpke syndrome*	Ulnar nerve muscles (finger flex/abduction), FDP (2nd, 3rd fingers), extensor pollicus longus/brevis (thumb extension/abduction)	Finger flexion
Lateral	Biceps, pronator teres, flexor carpi radialis	Biceps
Posterior	Latissimus dorsi, radial nerve hand (finger extension), deltoid (shoulder abduction)	Triceps
Medial	All ulnar innervated muscles (wrist finger flexion), & median innervated intrinsic hand muscles	Finger flexion

[1] *Erb-Duchenne syndrome*

Conus Medullaris or Cauda Equina Syndromes

Etiology: loss of spinal space due to trauma, central disc herniation at L3-S1, ankylosing spondylitis, rheumatoid arthritis, epidural hematoma or cancer. *Conus medullaris syndrome* has sudden onset with bilateral perineal and thigh pain. Motor loss is symmetric, mild fasciculations may be present, sensory loss is in saddle distribution, and bladder/rectal/sexual function is severely impaired. *Cauda equina syndromes* are gradual in onset, unilateral, with severe asymmetric pain in thighs, perineum, back and legs. Motor loss is asymmetric, severe and fasciculations are absent. Sensory loss is in saddle area and may be unilateral. Bladder/rectal/sexual functions have mild impairment. *Evaluate* with CT or MRI & consult spine surgeon.

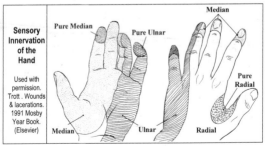

Sensory Innervation of the Hand

Used with permission. Trott . Wounds & lacerations. 1991 Mosby Year Book. (Elsevier)

Pure Median   Pure Ulnar   Median

Pure Radial

Median   Ulnar   Radial

Nerve	Motor Tests for Nerve Injury
Median	lie dorsum of hand on flat surface, palmar abduct thumb vs. resistance while palpating radial border of the thenar eminence (abd. pollicis brevis)
Ulnar	abduct fingers or pinch paper between thumbs, + prox. index fingers as pull in opposite direction. Nerve injury if thumb IP bends (*Froment's* sign)
Radial	extend fingers and wrist against resistance

Tendons of the Hand

Tendon	Test of Function (Nerves: M-median, R-radial, U-ulnar)
interossei	*Dorsal* (spread hand), *volar* (hold paper between fingers)(U)
lumbricals	Extend wrist + DIP/PIP as fingertips pressed down (M,U)
flexor dig. profundus	Flex DIP while MCP and PIP extended (M,U)
flexor dig. superficialis	Flex PIP while all other digits extended (M)
flexor dig. superficialis (of index finger)	Have thumb + index finger pinch or pick up. If FDS intact, DIP will hyperextend, If not intact, DIP will flex (M)
flex. carpi radialis/ulnaris	Flex and radially (M) or ulnar (U) deviate wrist
abd pollicis longus	Extension and abduction of thumb (R)
extensor pollicis brevis	Extension and abduction of thumb (R)
ext. carpi radialis longus	Make fist while extending wrist (R)
ext. carpi radialis brevis	Make fist while extending wrist (R)
ext. pollicis longus	Lift thumb off flat surface while palm is flat and down (R)
ext. digitorum communis	Extension of fingers at MCP joint (R)
ext. indicis proprius	Extension of index finger at MCP + other fingers in fist (R)
ext. digiti minimi	Extension of small finger while making a fist (R)
ext. carpi ulnaris	Extension and ulnar deviation of wrist (R)

dig. - digitorum, flex. - flexor, ext. - extensor, abd. - abductor DIP - distal interphalangeal joint, PIP - proximal interphalangeal joint, MCP - metacarpal phalangeal joint.

Compartment Syndromes

Etiology: ↓ in compartment size (e.g. crush) or ↑ in contents (e.g. swelling, bleed).

Symptoms	Compartment Pressures (CP)	
• Pain (esp. with passive movement)	• Normal	< 10 mm Hg
• Paresthesias (lose vibratory sense 1st)	• Abnormal	10-30 mm Hg
• Pallor or Pulselessness	• Compartment syndrome	> 30 mm Hg or MAP minus CP < 40 mm
• Paralysis		

Psychiatry

Folstein Mini-Mental Status Exam

Score	Orientation, Registration, Attention, Recall, Language/praxis
5	What is the year, season, date, day, month?
5	Where are we (city, state, country, hospital, floor)?
3	Name 3 objects: one second to say each. Ask patient for all 3 after you have said them. 1 point for each correct answer.
5	Serial 7s backward from 100 (stop after 5X) or spell WORLD backwards
3	Ask 3 objects above to be repeated. 1 point for each correct answer
2	Show pencil & watch and ask subject to name them
1	Ask patient to repeat "no ifs, ands, or buts."
3	Obey:"Take this paper in your right hand, fold in ½, put it on floor"
1	Read & obey written command: "Close your eyes"
1	Write any sentence with a noun, verb (sentence must be sensible)
1	Copy design below: Copy design must contain all angles and 2 must intersect

A score ≤ 23 is abnormal (organic brain syndrome)   *J Psychiat Res* 1975; 12: 189.

Differentiating Between Delirium, Dementia, and Acute Psychosis

Feature	Delirium	Dementia	Psychosis
Age of onset	Any	Usually older	13-40 years
Psychiatric history	Usually absent	Usually absent	Present
Emotion	Labile	Normal or labile	Flat affect
Vital signs	Abnormal	Normal	Normal
Onset	Sudden	Gradual	Sudden
24h course	Fluctuates	Stable	Stable
Consciousness	Altered ↓	Clear	Clear
Attention	Disordered	OK unless severe	Can be disordered
Cognition	Disordered	Impaired	Selective
Hallucinations	Visual or sensory	Rare	Auditory
Delusions	Fleeting	Rare	Sustained, grand
Orientation	Impaired	Often Impaired	Rarely impaired
Psychomotor	↑ or ↓ or Shifting	Normal	Variable
Speech	Incoherent	Perseveration, difficult find word	Normal, slow or rapid
Involuntary move	Asterixis or tremor	Often absent	Usually absent
Physical illness or drug toxicity	Drug toxicity	Either (esp. Alzheimer's)	Neither

Emerg Med Clin North Am 2000; 18: 243.

Final Diagnoses in ED Patients with NEW Psychiatric Complaints

Organic Disease		Functional/Psychiatric Disease	
Toxin ingestion/abuse	30%	Psychotic	17%
Dementia	7%	(not schizophrenia)	
Postictal	6%	Schizophrenia	13%
Metabolic (Ca, Na, glucose, O_2)	6%	Depressive disorders	3%
Infectious	5%	Other	4%
Other	9%		

Medical Evaluation of ED Patients with NEW Psychiatric Complaints[1,2]

Evaluation	Diagnostic	Evaluation	Diagnostic
• History	27%	Electrolytes with BUN,	
• Examination/O_2 sat.	6%	creatinine, glucose	10%
• Drug screen/alcohol	29%	CT scan	10%
• Complete blood count	5%	Lumbar puncture	8%

1. Above evaluation is indicated for new psychiatric complaints, with consideration of thyroid screen, CPK (to exclude rhabdomyolysis), CXR & a more focused (limited or expanded) evaluation based on history & exam. Most patients in cited study with meningitis or a positive LP had no fever.(Only 38% had LP performed) *Ann Emerg Med* 1994; 24: 673.
2. Others have found that patients with isolated psychiatric complaints and a prior history of psychiatric illness with normal examination, and normal vitals without medical complaints may be referred without ancillary ED testing. *J Emerg Med* 2000; 18: 173.

"Modified SAD PERSONS" Scale[1]

Factor	Points[1]
Sex (male)	1
Age less than 19 years OR above 45 years	1
Depression or hopelessness (admits to depression or ↓ concentration, appetite, sleep, or libido)	2
Previous suicide attempts or previous psychiatric care (in or outpatient)	1
Excess alcohol or drug use	1
Rational thinking lost (organic brain syndrome or psychosis)	2
Separated, divorced, or widowed	1
Organized or serious suicide attempt	2
No social support (close family, friend, job, active religious affiliation)	1
Stated future intent to harm self	2

1. Before discharging a depressed patient from the ED, make sure patient is not actively suicidal, has a support system at home, and has no firearms.
2. 0 – 5 total points – low probability (< 5%) of requiring psychiatric admission
  6 – 8 total points – intermediate probability (~ 50%) of requiring admission
  ≥ 9 total points – high probability (≥ 75%) of requiring admission

Upper Respiratory Infections

	Clinical Feature	Points	Total Score & (Strep. throat risk)
McIsaac modification of Centor score for Strep. pharyngitis	History of fever or temp >38°C	1	-1 or 0 (1%)
	Absence of cough	1	1 (10%)
	Tender anterior cervical nodes	1	2 (17%)
	Tonsillar swelling or exudates	1	3 (35%)
	Age < 15	1	4 (> 50%)
	Age ≥ 45	-1	5 (> 50%)

See page 93 for antibiotic recommendation   *JAMA* 2000; 284: 2912.

Diagnostic Tests

Alveolar-arterial Oxygen gradient (A-a gradient)

Formula: $(AP-47) \times FiO_2$ [150 room air at sea level] $- (paO_2 + pCO_2/0.8)$

(AP) Atmospheric pressure – mm Hg	Altitude (feet)	Atmospheric pressure - mm Hg	Altitude (feet)
760	Sea level (0 feet)	609	6,000
707	2,000	564	8,000
656	4,000	523	10,000

Normal A-a gradient = (Patient's age)/4 +4,
FiO_2 = fraction inspired oxygen (21% on room air at sea level)

Dead Space

VT = tidal volume; VDS_{aw} = airway dead space volume
$VD_{phys}/VT = (paCO_2 - pETCO_2)/paCO_2$ [$pETCO_2$ = mean end-tidal CO_2]
Alveolar dead space fraction = $V_{ADS}/VT = (VD_{phys}/VT - VDS_{aw}/VT) \times 100\%$
Modified dead space equation: $= 100 \times (PaCO_2 - PetCO_2)/PaCO_2$
Normal alveolar dead space fraction < 20%

Acute Asthma & Chronic Obstructive Pulmonary Disease (COPD)

Predicted PEFR[1] in Adult Females								
Height (in)	58	60	62	64	66	68	70	
Age (yr) 20	453	459	465	471	476	481	485	[1]PEFR = peak expiratory flow rate.
25	464	471	477	482	488	493	498	(Liters/min)
30	468	474	481	486	492	497	502	
35	468	474	480	485	491	496	501	
40	463	469	475	481	486	491	496	
50	446	452	458	463	469	474	478	*Br Med J* 1989
60	424	430	435	440	445	450	454	298: 1068-1070.

Predicted PEFR[1] in Adult Males							
Height (in)	63	65	67	69	71	73	75
Age (yr) 20	567	575	583	591	598	605	611
25	594	603	611	619	626	633	640
30	608	617	625	633	641	648	655
35	613	622	631	639	646	654	661
40	612	620	629	637	645	652	660
50	594	602	610	618	626	633	640
60	564	572	580	587	594	601	607

[1]PEFR = peak expiratory flow rate. (Liters/minute)

Br Med J 1989 298: 1068-1070.

Management Options in Acute Asthma

General	• Administer O_2 and apply cardiac monitor, pulse oximeter
Inhaled β_2 agonist	• Administer via nebulizer continuous or q30 min if moderate to severe **OR** via MDI 2-4 puffs q 4 hours if mild asthma • (1) albuterol (*Ventolin*) 2.5-5 mg or (2) levalbuterol (*Xopenex*) 0.63-1.25 mg
Anticholinergics	• ipratropium bromide (*Atrovent*): 0.5 mg in 2.5 ml NS via nebulizer • **OR** 4-8 puffs qid (18 µg /puff)
Steroids	• methylprednisolone (*Solu-Medrol*) 1-2 mg/kg IV (if cannot take PO) **OR** prednisone 1-2 mg/kg PO; continue X 5-7 days (do not taper) • Inhaled steroids (*Azmacort, Aerobid, Beclovent, Flovent, Vanceril*) after stopping oral steroids if frequent oral steroids or severe asthma
Other options	• Magnesium sulfate ($MgSO_4$) 2 g IV over 15 min if severe asthma and no renal failure • epinephrine 0.3 mg SC **OR** terbutaline 0.25 mg SC q 20 min X 2 • prophylaxis (not acute treatment) with oral zafirlukast (*Accolate*), montelukast (*Singulair*) or zileuton (*Zyflo*)

Criteria Predicting Severe Disease & Admission	• Pretreatment PEFR < 80L/min, FEV1 < 1L (25% predicted) • Posttreatment PEFR <200L/min, FEV1 <1.6L (60% predicted) • PEFR ↑< 15% after treatment (if initial PEFR < 80% predicted) • Posttreatment PEFR and FEV1 < 60% predicted or PO_2 <60-80, PCO_2 > 40-45, pH <7.35, or SaO_2 <93%

One study found that peak flow did not correlate with likelihood of relapse while a history of frequent ED visits (> 5 in prior year), a history of frequent urgent care visits (> 5 in prior year), home nebulizer use, > 23 hour to ≤ 7 day duration of symptoms prior to initial ED visit, and asthma triggers (10% increase in relapse rate for each trigger [e.g. cigarettes, upper respiratory infection, environmental allergen, exercise, reproductive & psychosocial triggers]) were associated with ED relapse.

Chest 1999; 115: 919.

Guidelines for ED Management of Asthma NIH. *Ann Emerg Med* 1998; 31: 579.

History, examination, O_2 saturation, peak flow (PEFR) or $FEV1$

FEV1 or PEFR > 50%	FEV1 or PEFR < 50%	Impending arrest
• β_2-agonist by MDI or neb. X 3 1st hr • O_2 to keep sat. ≥ 90 % • Oral steroids if no immediate response	• High dose β_2-agonist + anticholinergic neb q 20 min or continue X 1 hr • O_2 to keep sat. ≥ 90 % • PO steroids	• Intubation + ventilate with 100% • β_2-agonist + anti-cholinergic neb. • IV steroids

Repeat exam, PEFR, O_2 saturation as needed

Admit to ICU (see below)

Moderate exacerbation	Severe exacerbation
• PEFR 50-80% of predicted best • Moderate symptoms • Inhaled β_2-agonists q 60 minutes • PO or increased inhaled steroids • Treat 1-3 hours, if improvement	• PEFR < 50% of predicted best • Severe rest symptoms, high risk • No improvement after initial treatment • Inhaled β_2-agonists q1h or continuous and inhaled anticholinergics • O_2 and systemic steroids

Good response	Incomplete response	Poor response
• PEFR ≥ 70% X 60 min • Normal exam	• PEFR ≥ 50%, < 70% • ≤ moderate symptoms	• PEFR < 50%, severe • pCO_2 ≥ 42 mm Hg

OR ↓ (individualize)

Discharge home	Admit to hospital	Admit to ICU
• continue inhaled β_2-agonists + oral steroid • Patient education regarding medicines, review plan, follow-up	• Inhaled β_2-agonist and anticholinergic, O_2 • PO or IV steroid • O_2 to keep sat. ≥ 90 % • Follow PEFR,HR,O_2sat	• Inhaled β_2-agonist hourly or continuous • IV steroids, O_2 • Oxygen • Possible intubation

American Thoracic Society (ATS) COPD Guidelines

COPD ATS Disease Severity Scale	Individual features	Disease Severity
	Worsening dyspnea	Mild if 1 feature plus additional finding[1]
	↑sputum purulence	Moderate if 2 features
	↑sputum volume	Severe if 3 features

[1] URI in past 5 days, fever, increased (↑) wheezing or cough, ↑HR or RR by ≥ 20%

ATS Recommendations for Management of COPD Exacerbation

Useful	(1) Admit CXR [24% abnormal rate], (2) β agonists/anticholinergics – inhaled, (3) Steroids up to 2 weeks (4) oxygen cautiously if hypoxemia, (5) BiPAP, CPAP, (6) Narrow spectrum antibiotics (*Amoxil, Septra,* tetracycline) if outpatient, no pneumonia present
Not useful	(1) spirometry for severity assessment (2) mucolytics (3) chest physiotherapy, (4) methylxanthines (5) any risk stratification methods for predicting relapse or inpatient mortality.

American Thoracic Society. *Ann Intern Med* 2001;134: 595)

Noninvasive Positive Pressure Ventilation (NPPV)

Disease states amenable to NPPV	Clinical criteria for NPPV use
Acute respiratory failure (e.g ARDS, pneumonia, asthma/COPD, pulmonary edema, neuromuscular disease) Chronic respiratory failure Acute pulmonary edema Chronic congestive heart failure with breathing related sleep disorder	Moderate to severe respiratory distress • increased dyspnea, • respiratory rate >24, • accessory muscles, • paradoxic breathing $PaCO_2$ > 45 mmHg and pH < 7.35 $Pa0_2/Fio_2$ < 200
Relative contraindications for NPPV	
Failure at prior NPPV attempts Hemodynamic instability/GI bleed Life threatening arrhythmias High risk of aspiration Airway obstruction	Impaired mental status Inability to use nasal or face mask Life threatening refractory hypoxemia ($Pa0_2$ < 60 mm Hg with $Fi0_2$ = 1.0) pH < 7.20

New Engl J Med 1997; 337: 1746. & Comprehensive Resp Med. 1999 Mosby, Phil; 3.12

NPPV Modes/Parameters

Volume mechanical	Breaths of 250-500 ml (4-8 ml/kg), pressures vary
Pressure mechanical	Pressure support or pressure control at 8-20 cm H_20, End-expiratory pressure of 0-6 cm H_20, volumes vary
BiPAP	Inspiratory pressure of 8 (6-14 cm) H_20, End expiratory pressure of 4 (3-5 cm) H_20, volumes vary, initial RR = 8
CPAP	5-13 cm H_20, volumes vary
Weaning parameters for all NPPV modes	• Clinically stable for 4-6 hours • Respiratory rate < 24/minute & Heart rate < 110 • Compensated pH > 7.35 • $Sa0_2$ > 90-92%% on ≤ 3L face mask 0_2

New Engl J Med 1997; 337: 1746

Prediction of Mortality from Community Acquired Pneumonia (PORT score)

STEP ONE

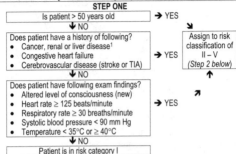

| Is patient > 50 years old | → YES |

↓ NO

Does patient have a history of following?
- Cancer, renal or liver disease[1]
- Congestive heart failure
- Cerebrovascular disease (stroke or TIA)   → YES

↓ NO

Does patient have following exam findings?
- Altered level of consciousness (new)
- Heart rate ≥ 125 beats/minute
- Respiratory rate ≥ 30 breaths/minute
- Systolic blood pressure < 90 mm Hg
- Temperature < 35°C or ≥ 40°C   → YES

↓ NO

Patient is in risk category I

Assign to risk classification of II – V *(Step 2 below)*

STEP TWO

Factor	Points	Factor	Points
Male age in years	age	Systolic BP ≤ 90 mmHg	+ 20
Female age in years	age – 10	Temp. < 35°C or ≥ 40°C	+ 15
Live in nursing home	+ 10	Heart rate ≥ 125/minute	+ 10
Neoplastic disease[1]	+ 30	Arterial pH < 7.35	+ 30
Liver disease[1]	+ 20	BUN 30 > mg/dl	+ 20
Congestive heart failure[1]	+ 10	Sodium < 130 mEq/L	+ 20
Cerebrovascular disease[1]	+ 10	Glucose ≥ 250 mg/dl	+ 10
Renal disease[1]	+ 10	Hematocrit < 30 g/dl	+ 10
Altered mentation	+ 20	PaO2 < 60 mm Hg	+ 10
Respirations ≥ 30/min	+ 20	Pleural effusion	+ 10

Add Points from Step 2 Above to Determine Risk Category, Total Points, and 30 Day Mortality[2,3]	Risk Category	Total Points	30 Day Mortality
	Class I	-	0.1 – 0.4%
	Class II	≤ 70	0.6 – 0.9%
	Class III	71 – 90	0.9 – 2.8%
	Class IV	91 – 130	8.5 – 9.3%
	Class V	> 130	27.0 – 31.1%

1 Neoplastic – any non skin basal/squamous skin cancer active or diagnosed in past year; Liver – liver histology (biopsy) or clinical exam evidence chronic hepatitis or cirrhosis; Cerebrovascular – any prior stroke or TIA; Renal – abnormal BUN/creatinine, Congestive heart failure – systolic or diastolic ventricular dysfunction documented by history, exam, CXR, Echo, MUGA scan or ventriculogram.

2 Class I – III. outpatient treatment, Class IV – admit to floor, Class V –ICU admit.

3 Use scoring system in conjunction with physician judgement. Patients with vomiting, no support system, immune defect, or O₂ Sat ≤ 90% may require admission despite low PORT score. (PORT). *N Engl J Med* 1997; 336: 243.; Clin Infect Dis 2000; 31: 347

Thromboembolism-Pulmonary Embolism (PE)-Deep Venous Thrombosis (DVT)

Pulmonary Emboli Risk Factors	Clinical Features	
• Immobility, Venous damage	Chest pain (pleuritic-75%)	80-90%
• Hypercoagulability (e.g. cancer, prior clot, nephrotic syndrome, inflammatory disease, recent pregnancy < 3 months), estrogens, sepsis, lupus,	Dyspnea	73-84%
	Cough (wheeze – 9%)	37-53%
	Hemoptysis	13-30%
	Respirations ≥ 16/min (≥ 20)	92(70%)
• No risk factors in 15% overall	Fever > 100° F/tachycardia	43/40%
• No risk factors in 28% < 40 years old	Calf swelling	30%

Diagnostic Studies	ECG Findings	
• <u>CXR</u> – abnormal in 60-84%	• Nonspecific ST-T changes	50%
• <u>Art. blood gas</u> – 92% ↑A-a gradient[1]	• T wave inversion	42%
• <u>Ventilation perfusion scan V/Q</u> – below	• New right bundle branch	15%
• <u>D-Dimer</u>- 85-95% sensitive	• S in 1,Q in 3, T in 3	12%
• <u>Angiography</u>- > 98% sensitive/specific	• Right axis deviation	7%
• <u>Echo</u> – detects 90% causing ↓BP	• Shift in transition to V5	7%
• <u>CT</u> - ~ 90% sensitive for central PE	• Right ventricle hypertrophy	6%
• <u>MRI</u> – > 90% sensitive for PE	• P pulmonale	6%

A-a gradient: 150 – (paO$_2$ + pCO$_2$/0.8); Normal = age/4 +4.

Charlotte Rule for Excluding Pulmonary Embolism (see rule application, page 135)

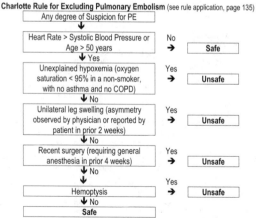

Charlotte Rule Application

Patients designated as **safe** have a 13.3% probability of having a PE. In the cited study, safe patients with either (1) a negative whole blood D-dimer (SimpliRED or SimpliFY) plus a normal dead space (< 20%, modified dead space = 100 X ($PaCO_2$ – $PetCO_2$)/$PaCO_2$) or (2) a quantitative D-dimer assay < 500 ng/ml were felt to have a low enough probability of PE that no further evaluation was necessary. If any of above tests are abnormal (any abnormal D-dimer or dead space ≥ 20%), then radiologic imaging (CT, V/Q or angiogram) is required.

Patients designated as **unsafe** have a 42% probability of having a PE. These patients require radiologic imaging (CT, V/Q, or angiogram) to exclude PE.

Ann Emerg Med 2002; 39: 144; & 2003; 42: 266.

Pulmonary Embolus - *Wicki* (Geneva) Clinical Probability Score

PE Probability[1]	Total	PE Probability[2]	Predictor	Points
Low (10%)	0	~ 4%	Age 60-79 years	+1
	1	~ 8%	Age ≥ 80 years	+2
	2	~ 7%	Prior PE or DVT	+2
	3	~ 10%	Recent surgery[3]	+3
	4	~ 17%	Heart rate > 100	+1
Intermediate (38%)	5	~ 22%	$PaCO_2$ < 36 mm Hg	+2
	6	~ 42%	$PaCO_2$ = 36 - 38.9 mm Hg	+1
	7	~ 43%	PaO_2 < 48.7 mm Hg	+4
	8	~ 55%	PaO_2 = 48.7 - 59.9 mm Hg	+3
High (81%)	9	~ 77%	PaO_2 = 60 - 71.1 mm Hg	+2
	10	~ 77%	PaO_2 = 71.1 - 82.3 mm Hg	+1
	11	~ 85%	Plate-like atelectasis	+1
	12	100%	Elevated hemidiaphragm	+1

[1] Aggregate and [2] Individual probability of pulmonary embolism based on total points
[3] Recent surgery = orthopedic, hip, knee, pelvic or abdominal surgery during prior month

Arch Intern Med 2001; 161: 92-97.

Pulmonary Embolus – *Well's* (Canadian) Clinical Probability Score

Criteria	Points	Total score (PE probability)
Suspected DVT	3	Low - < 2 total points
Other diagnosis less likely than PE	3	3.6 % probability of PE
Heart rate > 100	1.5	Moderate - 2-6 total points -
Immobile or surgery in prior 4 weeks	1.5	20.5% probability of PE
Prior DVT or PE	1.5	High - > 6 total points
Hemoptysis	1	66.7% probability of PE
Cancer (palliative, treated prior 6 mo)	1	*Thromb Haemost 2000; 83: 416.*

D dimer/Dead Space[1,2] Accuracy in Diagnosis of Pulmonary Embolism

Test	Sensitivity[3]	Specificity[3]	Negative LR[4]	Positive LR[4]
⊕ D dimer OR ⊕ Dead space	98.4 (92-100)	51.6 (46-57)	0.03	2.03
⊕ D dimer	93.4 (85-98)	67.1 (62-72)	0.09	2.85
⊕ Dead space	67.2 (53-77)	76.3 (72-81)	0.43	2.83

[1] Dead space calculation, see page 129 , [2] D-dimer test used in study = whole blood agglutination assay (e.g. SimpliRED), ELISA may be more accurate, [3] Diagnostic values with 95% confidence intervals listed, [4] LR – likelihood ratio *JAMA* 2001; 285: 761.

American College of Emergency Physicians
Clinical Policy in Suspected Pulmonary Embolism (PE) www.acep.org

Level	Specific Recommendations
Level A	• No level A recommendations for D-dimer testing alone • No level A recommendations for chest CT used alone • In patients with a low to moderate pretest probability of PE, a normal perfusion scan reliably exclude a clinically significant PE
Level B	• If low pretest probability of PE (1) a negative quantitative D-dimer assay (turbimetric or ELISA) or (2) a negative whole blood cell qualitative D-dimer assay & a Well's score < 2 (page 135) excludes PE. • If low to moderate pretest probability of PE and an indeterminate V/Q scan, one of the following tests can be used to exclude clinically significant PE: (1) a negative quantitative D-dimer assay (turbimetric or ELISA), (2) a negative whole blood cell qualitative D-dimer with a Well's score ≤ 4 (page 135), (3) a negative single bilateral venous US scan for low probability patients, (4) a negative serial bilateral venous US for moderate probability patients. • Thin collimation spiral thoracic CT with 1-2 mm image reconstruction may be used as an alternative to V/Q scan for suspected PE.
Level C	• If low pretest probability of PE, a negative whole blood D-dimer assay alone or immunofiltration D dimmer assay excludes PE. • If low to moderate pretest probability of PE and a nondiagnostic V/Q use a negative whole blood D-dimer assay to exclude PE. • Spiral CT of the thorax with delayed CT venography may be used for increased detection of significant PE.

Level A – generally accepted principles of management.
Level B – a range of strategies with moderate clinical certainty
Level C – strategies based on preliminary, inconclusive or conflicting evidence.

V/Q Result & Probability of Pulmonary Embolism

Clinical Suspicion	Ventilation-Perfusion Scan Result		
	Low probability[1]	Intermediate	High probability
Low	4%	16%	56%
High	40%	66%	96%

[1]If low prob scan+comorbidity, mortality = 8%. If no comorbidity, mortality = 0.15%.
Emerg Med Reports 1996; 119.

Management Options in Pulmonary Embolism

Heparin	• Load 80 U/kg, drip 18u/kg/hour IV, see page 138 for ongoing adjustment of heparin infusion
Thrombolytics	• <u>Indications (controversial)</u>: shock or significant respiratory distress or significant hypoxia.
	• <u>Dose</u>: (1) tPA 100 mg IV over 2 hours **OR** (2) streptokinase 250,000 U IV over 30 min, then 100,000 U/hour X 24 hours (administer infusion over 72 hours if concurrent deep venous thrombosis is suspected)
	• May be used up to 1-2 weeks after symptom onset
Vena Cava filter	• Indications: (1) strong contraindication to anticoagulation **OR** (2) clot develops while adequately anticoagulated
Embolectomy	• Indication: If not anticoagulation candidate & acutely unstable

Management of Suspected Pulmonary Embolism in Pregnancy

There is minimal fetal risk from performing a ventilation-perfusion scan or CT scan of the chest, while an undiagnosed pulmonary embolus can be deadly for both the mother and fetus. Keep Foley in to empty bladder and lessen fetal exposure during radiological imaging (CT, V/Q scan).

(1) Doppler (Duplex) legs	• If abnormal, treat patient. False positive Doppler studies can occur after 20 weeks gestation due to vena cava compression.
(2) D-dimer	• First trimester D-dimer > 700 ng/ml, 2nd trimester D-dimer > 1,000, and 3rd trimester D-dimer > 1,420 are abnormal.
	• Exact cut-off required for imaging/evaluation is undefined.
(3) Imaging Option 1 V/Q scan	• If Doppler normal, perform reduced dose perfusion scan after IV NS & Foley placed to empty dye from bladder. Normal = no PE.
	• Perform ventilation scan if perfusion scan is abnormal.
Imaging Option 2 CT	• Many experts feel that CT may deliver less radiation to the fetus than V/Q scan and feel that CT is appropriate radiological study if Doppler of lower extremities is normal.
Treatment	• Use heparin protocol above. Warfarin is contraindicated.

Radiology 2002; 224: 487.; *Acad Emerg Med* 2004; 11: 269.; *AJR* 2003; 1495.;

Clinical Estimate of the Probability of DVT (total points)[1,2]

Active cancer (or treated past 6 mo)	1	Calf > 3 cm larger than other side[3]	1
Paralysis, paresis, recent leg cast	1	Pitting edema, greater in one leg	1
Entire leg swollen	1	Collateral superficial veins	
Tender along deep venous system	1	(nonvaricose)	1
Recent bed-ridden for > 3 days or major surgery within 4 weeks	1	Alternative diagnosis as likely or greater than that of DVT	-2

1 *High* probability (75% DVT prevalence) if score ≥ 3; *Moderate* probability (17% DVT) if
  score = 1 or 2; *Low* probability (3% DVT) if score ≤ 0.
2 Score is not useful if prior thromboembolism, suspect pulmonary embolus, pregnancy, or
  patient taking warfarin.
3 Measure 10 cm below tibial tuberosity.   *JAMA* 1998; 279: 1094.

Evaluation of Suspected DVT Based on Pretest Probability (PTP)- see above

Low PTP Doppler Ultrasound		Moderate PTP Doppler Ultrasound (US)		High PTP Doppler Ultrasound	
Normal	Abnormal[1]	Normal	Abnormal	Normal	Abnormal
↓	↓	↓	↓	↓	↓
No DVT	venogram	Repeat US In 1 week	Treat DVT	venogram	Treat DVT
	↙ ↓	↓ ↘		↓ ↘	
Abnormal	Normal	Normal	Abnormal	Normal	Abnormal
Treat DVT	No DVT	No DVT	Treat DVT	No DVT	Treat DVT

1 some experts would treat instead of obtaining venogram   *JAMA* 1998; 279: 1094.

Weight Based Nomogram for Dosing Heparin

Heparin 80 U/kg IV, then 18 U/kg/hour. Measure PTT q6h. Adjust dose as follows:

Measured PTT	Heparin Adjustment
< 35 sec (1.2 X control)	• 80 U/kg bolus, then ↑rate by 4 U/hour
35-45 sec (1.2 - 1.5 X control)	• 40 U/kg bolus, then ↑rate by 2 U/hour
46-70 sec (1.5 - 2.3 X control)	• No change
71-90 sec (2.3 - 3 X control)	• ↓ rate by 2 U/kg/hour
> 90 sec (3 X control)	• stop infusion X 1 h, then ↓rate by 3 U/kg/h

Chest 2001; 119.

Low Molecular Weight (LMW) Heparin for DVT

• Comparable safety (with less occurrence of thrombocytopenia) compared to
  standard unfractionated heparin has been found.

• Regimens (*Lovenox*) –1 mg/kg SC bid or 1.5 mg/kg SC q 24h
    - Enoxaparin (*Lovenox*) –1 mg/kg SC bid or 1.5 mg/kg SC q 24h
    - Dalteparin (*Fragmin*) – 100-120 U/kg SC bid or 200 U/kg SC q 24h

• Begin either (LMW) heparin regimen in addition to warfarin on same day. INR
  should be 2.0 - 3.0 for at least two days before discontinuing LMW heparin.

• Contraindications – major bleed risk, poor compliance/follow-up, renal failure.
                        Mayo Clin Proc 1998; 73: 545; *N Engl J Med* 1996; 335: 1816.

American College of Emergency Physicians
Clinical Policy in Suspected Deep Venous Thrombosis (DVT)

Level	Specific Recommendations[1]
Level A	• No level A recommendations for D-dimer testing alone • No level A recommendations for lower extremity ultrasound used alone
Level B	• If low pretest probability, DVT can be excluded by (1) a negative quantitative D-dimer assay (turbimetric or ELISA) or (2) a negative whole blood cell qualitative D-dimer plus a low probability DVT score (see above) or (3) a negative whole blood D-dimer alone for proximal DVT only • If low pretest probability of DVT, a negative single venous ultrasound (US) excludes proximal lower extremity DVT, and clinically significant distal DVT. • If moderate to high pretest probability of DVT, serial venous US need to be performed. • If high suspicion of pelvic or inferior vena thrombosis suspected, additional imaging may be required (e.g. MRI pelvis)
Level C	• Consider fibrinolytic therapy in patients with limb threatening thrombosis of the iliofemoral system in whom benefits of treatment outweigh risks of serious bleeding complications.

Level A – generally accepted principles of management.

Level B – a range of strategies with moderate clinical certainty

Level C – strategies based on preliminary, inconclusive or conflicting evidence.

www.acep.org

Seizures and Status Epilepticus

Status epilepticus – Continuous seizure for ≥ 30 minutes or ≥ 2 seizures without full recovery of consciousness between seizures.

Most Common Causes of Status Epilepticus in Adults

Etiology	Percent[1]
• Anticonvulsant withdrawal	25%
• Alcohol withdrawal	25%
• Cerebrovascular (stroke, anoxia, and hemorrhage)	22%
• Metabolic (encephalopathy due to low glucose, or infection)	22%
• Trauma	15%
• Drug toxicity (see page 144 for drugs that cause seizures)	15%
• Central nervous system infection	12%
• Central nervous system tumor or congenital CNS lesion (8% each)	8%
• Prior epilepsy	33%
• Idiopathic – no cause is found	30%

[1] Total adds up to > 100% due to multiple causes   *Neurol Clin North Am* 1998;16:257

Seizure Management

1. Protect airway, administer O_2, start IV, attach cardiac monitor and pulse oximeter, and prepare intubation equipment.
2. Perform stat bedside glucose test, send electrolytes and drug levels.
3. Administer D_{50} 1 amp IV if hypoglycemia, and thiamine 100 mg if malnourished.
4. Intravenous drug therapy as per table. If the first drug is unsuccessful, try another agent. If this is unsuccessful, consider general anesthesia.
5. Treat fever and correct sodium, calcium, or magnesium abnormalities.

Intravenous Drug Therapy for Status Epilepticus[1]

	Drug	Dose & route	Maximum rate	Special features
A	lorazepam	0.1 mg/kg IV	2 mg/min	may repeat q5min x2
	or diazepam	0.15 mg/kg IV	5 mg/min	may repeat q5min x2
	or diazepam	0.2 mg/kg PR	--	may repeat dose x1
B	fosphenytoin[2]	15-18 mg/kg IV	< 150 mg/min	monitor closely
	or phenytoin	20 mg/kg IV	< 50 mg/min	
C	phenobarbital	15-30 mg/kg IV	50-75 mg/min	monitor closely
D	pentobarbital (coma)	10-15 mg/kg (load)	slow IV	intubation required;
		0.5-1.0 mg/kg/h	< 50 mg/min	vasopressors prn
E	midazolam drip	0.1-0.3 mg/kg IV	< 1-2 mg/min	respiratory and blood pressure depression
		0.075-10 micrograms/kg/h		

[1] If toxin ingested and status epilepticus, also manage as per specific toxin overdose.
[2] Dose in fosphenytoin PE (phenytoin equivalents) – administer at rate of < 150 mg/min.

Surgical Abdominal Disorders

Diagnoses in ED patients > 65 y with Acute Abdominal Pain (≤ 1 week)

Physicians should have a low threshold for surgical consultation and admission/observation in elderly patients with undiagnosed abdominal pain.

Pain of unknown etiology	23%	Incarcerated hernia	4%
Biliary colic, cholecystitis	12%	Pancreatitis, UTI, volvulus, abscess	
Small bowel obstruction	12%	constipation, medications	Each 2%
Gastritis	8%	Aneurysm, ischemic bowel, hiatal	
Perforated viscus	7%	hernia, herpes zoster,	
Diverticulitis	6%	reducible hernia, myocardial	
Appendicitis	4%	infarction, pulmonary embolus	
Renal colic	4%	colon obstruction	Each < 1%

Ann Emerg Med 1990; 1383.

Appendicitis (MANTRELS diagnostic score)

Item	Score		Total	Action
Migration of pain to RLQ	1		≥ 7	Candidates for surgery
Anorexia or acetone in urine	1		4-6	Serial exams or further
Nausea with vomiting	1			testing is needed
Tenderness in right low quadrant	2			(e.g. CT or US)
Rebound tenderness	1			
Elevated temperature > 100.4 F	1		< 4	Extremely low probability
Leukocytosis; WBC > 10,500	2			of appendicitis, rare
Shift of WBC's; >75% neutrophils	1			cases have been < 4

MANTRELS score is less accurate in women compared to men. Therefore, it may be appropriate to obtain a CT or US in women with high scores. *Res Staff Phys* 1995; 11-18.

Biliary Tract Disease (Biliary Colic)

Clinical Features - Biliary Colic	Management of Biliary Colic
• Pain duration < 6-8 hours • Absence of fever • WBC < 11,000 cells/mm³ in most • Normal liver function tests in 98% • US is >98% sensitive for gallstones	• Treat pain • Anticholinergics (e.g. dicyclomine [Bentyl], atropine) are no more effective than placebo for pain relief. • Surgery follow up

Acute Cholecystitis

Clinical Features - Acute Cholecystitis		Management of Acute Cholecystitis
Pain duration > 6-8 hours	> 90%	• Exclude complications by US or CT
Temperature ≥ 100.4° F	25%	(e.g. choledocholithiasis, acute
Murphy's sign	> 95%	pancreatitis in 15%, gallstone ileus)
WBC > 11,000 cells/mm³	65%	• Treat pain
Elevated liver function tests	55%	• Administer antibiotics (page 87)
Ultrasound sensitivity	85%	• IV NS and take nothing by mouth

Ann Emerg Med 1996; 28: 273,& 278. *Ann Emerg Med* 1993; 22: 1363.

Mesenteric Ischemia

Causes: arterial embolus in 25-50% (esp. to superior mesenteric artery), arterial thrombosis 12-25%, venous thrombosis (esp. coagulopathy) + low cardiac output.
Risk factors: age, vascular/valvular disease, dysrhythmias, CHF, recent MI, hypovolemia, diuretics, β blockers splanchnic vasoconstrictor (e.g. digoxin).

Clinical Features		Diagnostic Studies	
• Abdominal pain	80-90%	• Elevated lactate	70-90%
• Sudden onset pain	60%	• WBC > 15,000 cells/mm^3	60-75%
• Vomiting	75%	• Elevated LDH	70%
• Diarrhea (often heme +)	40%	• Elevated CK	63%
• Gross GI bleeding	25%	• Elevated phosphate	30-65%
• _Early_: ↑pain with minimal abdominal tenderness	variable	• Plain xray – obstruction	30%
• _Late_: shock, fever confusion, distension, rebound, rigidity	variable	• Plain xray– thumb printing portal gas, or free air	< 20%
		• CT, US sensitivity	<50-70%
		• Angiography sensitivity	> 95%

Management
• Fluid and blood resuscitation
• Broad spectrum antibiotics (page 87)
• Surgical consult + emergency laparotomy (esp. if bowel necrosis, perforation)
• Mesenteric arteriography will demonstrate thrombosis, emboli, and mesenteric vasoconstriction and allow for selective papaverine administration until symptoms gone or surgery performed.
• Avoid digoxin & vasopressors due to vasoconstriction.

Emerg Med Clin North Am 1996; 571

Pancreatitis

Causes: gallstones, alcohols, drugs (table), infections (e.g. viral, Mycoplasma, Legionella, Ascaris, Salmonella), trauma, ↑ calcium, high triglycerides and certain metabolic disorders.

Clinical features – Epigastric pain radiating to back ± vomiting. Abdomen may be only mildly tender as pancreas is a retroperitoneal organ.

Complications: ↓Ca^{+2}, ↑glucose, ARDS, renal failure, bowel perforation, sepsis, pseudocyst or abscess formation, bleeding and death.

Select Drugs Causing Pancreatitis	
Definite	Probable
azathioprine	acetaminophen
cisplatin, ddl	cimetidine
furosemide	diphenoxylate
l-asparginase	estrogen
tetracycline	indomethacin
thiazides	mefenamic acid
sulfonamides	opiates
pentamidine	valproic acid

Diagnostics - Serum amylase is ↑ in 90-95% with acute pancreatitis. Many diseases cause hyperamylasemia (e.g. salivary gland & abd disorders, pregnancy renal failure, burns, alcoholism, DKA, pneumonia). If amylase ≥ 2-3 X normal, specificity is > 95%. ↑ lipase is more specific than ↑ amylase for pancreatitis.

Prognostic Signs in Pancreatitis[1]	
On admission[1]	In 48 hours[1]
Age > 55 y (70 y)	hematocrit fall > 10%
WBC > 16,000 (18k)	BUN rise > 5 mg/dl (>2)
glu > 200 mg/dl (220)	calcium < 8 mg/dl
LDH > 350 IU/L (400)	PaO_2 < 60 mm Hg
AST > 250 U/L	base deficit > 4mEq/L (>5)
	fluid sequestration > 6L(>4)

Mortality: < 1% if < 3, 25% if 3/4, 40% if 5/6, and 100% if > 6 prognostic signs listed above.

[1]Criteria for gallstone pancreatitis in parentheses

Computed Tomography Grading of Acute Pancreatitis

Grade	CT Findings	Abscess[1]	Mortality
A	Normal CT examination	0%	0%
B	Pancreatic enlargement alone	0%	0%
C	Inflammation of pancreas and peripancreatic fat	12%	0%
D	One peripancreatic fluid collection	17%	8%
E	≥ 2 peripancreatic fluid collections	61%	17%

[1]Rate of abscess formation   *Ann Surg* 1985;201:656; *N Engl J Med* 1994;330:1198.

Diagnostic Studies	Management
• Suspect abscess, hemorrhage, or pseudocyst if fever, persistent ↑ amylase, mass, ↑ bilirubin, ↑ WBC • US - 60-80% sensitive, 95% specific • CT - 90% sensitive, 100% specific • Obtain CT or US if suspect pseudocyst, abscess, gallstones or trauma	• IV fluids and narcotics prn • NG tube if persistent vomiting • If do not improve after 1 week, rule out abscess, pseudocyst, or ascites. • Surgery if: gallstones, bleeding, abscess, pseudocyst > 4 cm, deteriorate despite supportive care

N Engl J Med 1994; 330: 1198.

Toxins that Affect Vitals Signs and Physical Examination

Hypotension			Hypertension
ACE inhibitors	Antidepressants	Nitroprusside	Amphetamines
α & β antagonists	Disulfiram	Opioids	Anticholinergics
Anticholinergics	Ethanol, methanol	Organophosphates	Cocaine, Lead
Arsenic (acutely)	Iron, Isopropanol	Phenothiazines	MAO inhibitors
Ca^{+2} channel block	Mercury, GHB	Sedatives	Phencyclidine
Clonidine, cyanide	Nitrates	Theophylline	Sympathomimetics

Tachycardia			Bradycardia
Amphetamines	Ethylene glycol, iron		Antidysrhythmics
Anticholinergics	Organophosphates		α agonists, β antagonists
Arsenic (acutely)	Sympathomimetics		Ca^{+2} channel blockers
Antidepressants	PCP, Phenothiazines		Digitalis, opioids, GHB
Digitalis, disulfiram	Theophylline		Organophosphates

Tachypnea			Bradypnea
Ethylene glycol	Salicylates	Barbiturates	Isopropanol
Methanol	Sympathomimetics	Botulism	Opioids
Nicotine	(cocaine)	Clonidine	Organophosphates
Organophosphates	Theophylline	Ethanol	Sedatives

Hyperthermia			Hypothermia
Amphetamines	Phencyclidine		Carbon monoxide
Anticholinergics	Phenothiazines		Ethanol
Arsenic (acute)	Salicylates		Hypoglycemic agents
Cocaine	Sedative-hypnotics		Opioids
Antidepressants	Theophylline		Phenothiazines
LSD	Thyroxine		Sedative-hypnotics

Mydriasis (pupillodilation)			Miosis (pupilloconstriction)
Anticholinergics	Amphetamines	Anticholinesterase	Clonidine
Antihistamines	Cocaine	Opioids	Coma from barbit-
Antidepressants	Sympathomimetics	Nicotine	urates, benzodi-
Anoxia(any cause)	Drug withdrawal	Pilocarpine	azepines, ethanol

Toxins that Cause Seizures

Antidepressants	Cocaine, camphor	INH, Lead, Lithium	Organophosphates
β blockers	Ethanol withdrawal	PCP, theophylline	Sympathomimetics

[1]All agents causing ↓BP, fever, hypoglycemia and CNS bleeding can cause seizures.

Identification of Abused Drug Based on Street Name

Street name	Drug[1]	Street name	Drug[1]	Street name	Drug[1]
1 & 1	T + tri, T + Rit, Rit + V,	Jamestown	Jimsonweed	Shrooms	Psilocybe
		Jet	Ketamine	Silent partnr	Heroin
Acid	LSD	John Hinckly	PCP	Sinsemilla	Marijuana
Angel dust	LSD	Joy stick	MJ + PCP	Smack	Heroin
Apples	MJ	Juice	PCP	Snow-candy	Cocaine
Bam	H + Preludin	Junk	Heroin	Snort/nuff	Cocaine
Bazooka	Cocaine	Ketamine		Special LA	Ketamine
Bazooka paste	MJ+procaine	green/purpl	LSD	Speckld bird	Lookalike A
Bennies	A	Lady	Cocaine	Speed	A or M
Black beauty	CaffeinePPA	Loads	Cod + glu	Speedball	H + C
Black Molly	lookalike A	Love (ly)	PCP	Stardust	Cocaine
Blue Angels	A	Loveboat	MJ + PCP	Stuff	Heroin
Boat	PCP	Mauve	Ketamine	Super grass	PCP
Breakin'	Heroin	Maze	Fentanyl	SuperC or K	Ketamine
Brick	MJ	Mex. Maid	Heroin	Syrup&bean	Cod + V
Butt Naked	PCP	Mcky Mouse	LSD	T's & Blues	T + tri
Chiva	HMB	Monster	M	T's & Purple	T/tri/Narcan
Christmas trees	Depressant or stimulant	Mr. Natural	LSD	Tar	Opium
		Mud	H/molasses	Thriller	Heroin
Clickers	MJ + PCP	NASA	Heroin	Tic & Tac	PCP
Coast	Ritalin IV	Newboy	Heroin	Toot	Cocaine
Coke (Cola)	Cocaine	Nose candy	Cocaine	Tootsie roll	HMB
Crack	Rock C	Packs	Cod + glu	Tolley	Toluene
Crank	A, H, or M	Pasta	Cocaine	Unicorn	LSD
Crystal	M	Perks	Percdan/cet	USDA	Heroin
Disco hits	PCP	Peruvnwhite	Cocaine	Vitamin C	Cocaine
Dishrag	Heroin	Persia white	Fentanyl	WACs	MJ/blackflag roach killer
Dollies	Methadone	Pink & Grey	Darvon		
Dust (ed)	PCP	Pinkhearts	Lookalike A	Wack	PCP
Eve	Ecstasy	President	Heroin	Watergate	Heroin
4 & doors	Cod + glu	Purple	Ketamine	West Coast	Rit IV
Footballs	A	Risking high	Heroin	Whippet	Nitrousoxide
Girl	Cocaine	Robin's egg	Lookalike A	White(dust)	Cocaine
Green	Ketamine	Rock	A or M	White, China	Fentanyl
Happy dust	Cocaine	Roofies	Flunitrazepm	Window	
Happy sticks	MJ + PCP	Scat/Skag	Heroin	pane	LSD
Hawaiian wood rose	PCP	Shermans/ Sherms	PCP + MJ or formaldhyd	Wizard	LSD
				Yo Yo	Yohimbine

A (Amphetamines), C (Cocaine), Cod (codeine), glu (glutethemide), H (Heroin), Heroin – Mexican Brown (HMB), Marijuana (MJ), M (Methamphetamines), Rit (Ritalin), T (Talwin), tri (tripelennamine), V (Valium).

Toxidromes

Syndrome	Toxin	Manifestations
anticholinergic	*Natural*: belladonna alkaloids, atropine, homatropine, amanita muscurina. *Synthetics*: cyclopentolate, dicyclomine, tropicamide, antihistamines, tricyclics, phenothiazines	*Peripheral antimuscarinic*: delirium, dry skin, thirst, blurred vision, mydriasis, ↑ HR, ↑ BP, red rash, ↑ temperature, abdominal distention, urine retention. *Central symptoms*: delirium, ataxia, cardiovascular collapse, seizures
acetylcholinesterase inhibition	insecticides (organophosphates, carbamates)	*Muscarinic effects* (SLUDGE): salivation, lacrimation, urination, defecation, GI upset, emesis. Also ↓ or ↑ pulse and BP, miosis. *Nicotinic effects*: ↑ pulse, muscle fasciculations, weakness, paralysis, ↓ RR, sympathetic stimulation. *Central effects*: anxiety, ataxia, seizure, coma, ↓ respirations, cardiovascular collapse
cholinergic	acetylcholine, betelnut, bethanechol, Clitocybe, methacholine, pilocarpine	see *muscarinic* and *nicotinic* effects above
extrapyramidal	haloperidol, phenothiazines	*Parkinsonism*: dysphonia, rigidity, tremor, torticollis, opisthotonos
hemoglobinopathy	carbon monoxide, methemoglobin	headache, nausea, vomiting, dizziness, coma, seizures, cyanosis, cutaneous bullae, "chocolate" blood with methemoglobinemia
metal fume fever	fumes of iron, Mg, mercury, nickel, zinc, cadmium, copper	chills, fever, muscle pain, headache, fatigue, weakness
narcotic	morphine, dextromethorphan, heroin, fentanyl, meperidine, propoxyphene, codeine, diphenoxylate	CNS depression, miosis (except meperidine), ↓ respirations, ↓ BP, seizures (with propoxyphene and meperidine)
sympathomimetic	aminophylline, amphetamines, cocaine, ephedrine, caffeine, methylphenidate	CNS excitation, seizures, ↑ pulse, ↑ BP (↓ BP with caffeine)
withdrawal syndromes	alcohol, barbiturates, benzodiazepines, opioids	diarrhea, mydriasis, piloerection, ↑ BP, ↑ pulse, insomnia, lacrimation, cramps, yawning, hallucinations

Poisoning Antidotes and Treatments

Toxin	Antidote/Treatment	Other considerations
acetamino-phen	n-acetylcysteine see page 150 for dose	very effective if used within 8h, may be helpful up to 72h
β-blockers	Glucagon 1-5 mg IV/SC/IM (drip may be required)	glucagon may help reverse ↓pulse and ↓BP
Ca^{+2}channel blockers	CaCl$_2$ (10%) 10 ml IV, gluca-gon 1-5 mg IV/SC/IM	glucagon may help reverse ↓pulse and ↓BP
cyanide	*Lilly Cyanide Kit* (amyl nitrate, sodium nitrite, and sodium thiosulfate)	Treatment induces methemo-globinemia and ↓BP. Sodium thiocyanate is excreted in urine
digoxin	digoxin Fab fragments	see page 156 for dose
ethylene glycol	fomepizole (*Antizol*) – see page 166, 167	If fomepizole not available. Ethanol: goal is level of 0.1 g/dl. See Methanol page 167
isoniazid	pyridoxine 4 g IV, then 1 g IM q 30 min if needed	reverses seizures
methanol	fomepizole, ethanol, dialysis	also thiamine and folate
nitrites	methylene blue (0.2 ml/kg of 1% solution IV over 5 min)	consider exchange transfusion if severe methemoglobinemia
opiates	naloxone 0.4-2.0 mg IV,	diphenoxylate and propoxyphene may require higher doses
organo-phosphates, carbamates	atropine 0.05 mg/kg IV pralidoxime (PAM)	exceptionally high atropine doses may be necessary; PAM doesn't work for carbamate toxicity
salicylates	dialysis, or sodium bicarbonate 1 mEq/kg IV	goal of alkaline diuresis is serum pH of 7.50-7.55
tricyclic anti-depressants	sodium bicarbonate 1 mEq per kg IV (see text)	goal is serum pH of 7.50-7.55 to alter protein binding

Radio-opaque ingestions (CHIPES)	Drugs Cleared by Hemodialysis[1]	
• Chloral hydrate,chlorinated hydrocarbon • Heavy metals (arsenic, Pb, mercury) • Health food (bone meal, vitamins) • Iodides, iron • Potassium, psychotropics (e.g. phenothiazines, antidepressants) • Enteric coated tabs (KCl, salicylates) • Solvents (chloroform, CCl$_4$)	• Bromide • Salicylates • Lithium • Methanol	• Isopropyl alcohol • Chloral hydrate • Ethylene glycol
	Drugs cleared by Hemoperfusion[1]	
	• Barbiturates (e.g. phenobarbital) • Theophylline, Phenytoin • Possibly digoxin	

[1] Consult local poison center for more detail concerning latest indications

HAZMAT (Hazardous Materials)

Phone Numbers to Identify Hazardous Chemical Agents/Spills & their Management

• CDC/Agency for Toxic Substances Disease Registry (ATDSR). 404-488-7100

• Chemical Manufacturer's Association (CHEMTREC) 800-424-9300

General Approach to Poisoning

• Treat airway, breathing and BP	• Consider dextrose - 50 ml of D₅₀, naloxone 2 mg IV, and thiamine 100 mg IV
• Insert IV and apply cardiac monitor	
• Apply pulse oximeter, administer O_2	

Charcoal

According to the American Academy of Clinical Toxicology & European Association of Poison Centres and Clinical Toxicologists, single-dose activated charcoal should not be administered routinely in the management of poisoned patients. Based on volunteer studies, the effectiveness of activated charcoal decreases over time and the greatest benefit is within the 1ˢᵗ hour of ingestion. Administration of charcoal may be considered if a patient has ingested a potentially toxic amount of a poison (which is known to be adsorbed to charcoal) up to 1 hour previously. There are insufficient data to support or exclude its use after 1 hour of ingestion. There is no evidence that the administration of activated charcoal improves clinical outcome. Unless a patient has an intact or protected airway, the administration of charcoal is contraindicated.

Dose: initial dose is 1 g/kg PO or per NG mixed with cathartic such as sorbitol

Contraindications	Drugs Cleared by Multi-dose Charcoal[1]
• Unprotected airway • Corrosives, caustics (acids, alkalis) • Ileus, bowel obstruction • Drugs bound poorly by charcoal (arsenic, bromide, K⁺, toxic alcohols, heavy metals [iron, iodide, lithium])	theophylline, phenobarbital, digoxin, dextropropoxyphene, nadolol, phenytoin, diazepam, tricyclic antidepressants, chlorpropamide, nonsteroidals, and salicylates

[1] Administer repeat charcoal doses q 3-4 hours (use cathartic only for 1ˢᵗ dose).

Cathartics[1]

There are no definite indications for the use of cathartics in the management of the poisoned patient. If used, a cathartic should be limited to a single dose in order to minimize adverse effects.

Overview: Cathartics theoretically help by ↑ fecal elimination of charcoal-bound toxins, and preventing concretions. Monitor electrolytes closely with their use.

Contraindications	Cathartic choices
• Bowel injury, obstruction, perforation, or recent abdominal surgery • Hypotension, electrolytes abnormal (no magnesium if renal failure) • Corrosive or caustic ingestion	• Sorbitol (35-70%) – 1 g/kg PO/NG • Magnesium citrate 4 ml/kg PO or NG • Na⁺ or $MgSO_4$ – 250 mg/kg PO or NG

[1] Cathartics have never been shown to alter the clinical outcome in acute overdose.

Ipecac

There are insufficient data to support or exclude ipecac administration soon after poison ingestion. Based on experimental and clinical studies, ipecac should be considered only in an alert patient who has ingested a potentially toxic amount of a poison and if it can be administered within 60 minutes of the ingestion. Even then, clinical benefit has not been confirmed. (www.aactox.org)

	Absolute contraindications to ipecac
There are no absolute indications for ED use. Ipecac (30 ml PO) delays charcoal administration, incompletely empties the stomach and has many side effects.	• Unprotected airway • Pure caustics or hydrocarbons • Drugs that cause seizures, ↓mental status, ↓HR, or ↓respirations

Gastric lavage

Gastric lavage should not be considered unless a patient has ingested a potentially life-threatening amount of poison and the procedure can be performed < 60 min. after ingestion. Clinical benefit has not been confirmed in controlled studies.

Directions for Lavage in Overdose	_Indications_
• Use 36-40 French _Ewald_ tube • Lavage stomach with 250-300 ml NS or H_2O aliquots until the return is clear • Protect the airway with endotracheal intubation if there is an absent gag reflex, or altered mental status • Monitor the total input and output from the _Ewald_ tube to ensure fluid overload does not occur.	• Dangerous ingestion within 1 hour • Toxins that slow GI transit • Toxins with possible rapid onset seizure, or ↓mental status • Toxins poorly bound by charcoal
	Contraindications
	• Caustics (acids, alkalis), solvents (hydrocarbons), nontoxic ingestions, coagulopathy, GI tract pathology.

Whole bowel irrigation (WBI)

There are no absolute indications for WBI. WBI is an option for potentially toxic ingestions of sustained-release or enteric-coated drugs. WBI has theoretical value for patients who have ingested substantial amounts of iron or for the removal of ingested packets of illicit drugs and in the management of patients who have ingested substantial amounts of poisons not adsorbed to activated charcoal.

Administration	_Indications_
• Administer PO or place NG tube • Administer polyethylene glycol (_Go-Litely_) at 1-2 L/hour • Stop when objects recovered or • Stop when effluent clear	• Iron, zinc, Li, sustained release meds • Ingested crack vials or drug packets
	Contraindications
	• CNS or respiratory depression[1] • GI tract pathology (e.g. bleed, ileus, perforation, or obstruction)

[1] Unless intubated

Acetaminophen Toxicity

Phase	Time after ingestion	Signs and Symptoms
1	30 min to 24 hours	Asymptomatic, or minor GI irritant effects
2	24-72 hours	Relatively asymptomatic, GI symptoms resolve, possible mild elevation of LFT's or renal failure
3	72-96 hours	Hepatic necrosis with potential jaundice, hepatic encephalopathy, coagulopathy, and renal failure
4	4 days - 2 weeks	Resolution of symptoms or death

Acetaminophen

Ingestion of $\geq$ 140 mg/kg is potentially toxic. Obtain acetaminophen level $\geq$ 4h after acute ingestion and plot on the Rumack-Matthews nomogram. A 4h level $\geq$ 140 ug/ml indicates need for n-acetylcysteine. On nomogram (page 151), levels above dotted line (---------) indicates probable risk, while levels above the bottom solid line (_____) indicate possible risk of toxicity. If time from ingestion unknown, obtain level at time 0 and 4 h later to calculate half-life. If half-life is > 4 h, administer antidote.

Management	
Decontamination	<ul><li>Charcoal is indicated only if toxic co-ingestants are present.</li><li>Increase oral *Mucomyst* dose by 20% if charcoal given.</li></ul>
N-acetylcysteine N[AC] *Mucomyst* (*Acetadote* – IV formulation)	<ul><li>Assess toxicity based on nomogram.</li><li>If drug level will return in < 8 h post ingestion, treatment can be delayed until level known. NAC prevents 100% of toxicity if administered < 8 hours from ingestion. If level will return > 8 hours and $\geq$140 mg/kg ingested, administer 1st dose of *Mucomyst*. NAC is definitely useful $\leq$ 24 hours after ingestion, possibly up to 72 hours.</li><li>**PO Dose**: 140 mg/kg PO, then 70 mg/kg q4h X 17 doses. Shorter course (36 h) may be effective if no liver toxicity at 36 h. Contact poison center for short protocol specifics.</li><li>**IV Dose** - 150 mg/kg IV (in 200 ml D_5W) over 15 minutes, then 50 mg/kg (in 500 ml D_5W) over 4 hours, then 100 mg/kg (in 1000 ml D_5W) over 16 hours. Up to 18% develop anaphylactoid reaction (esp. if asthmatic or if prior NAC reaction). If this happens, discontinue and manage symptoms (e.g. antihistamines, epinephrine, inhaled ß agonists, IV fluids). If symptoms stop and were mild, consider restarting NAC. Otherwise, do not restart.</li></ul>

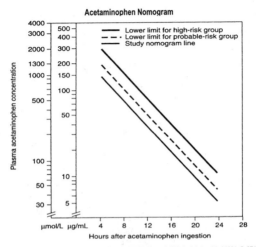

Acetaminophen Nomogram

Used with permission. Copyright 1981 AMA. Rumack BH. *Arch Intern Med* 1981; 5: 871.

βeta-Blockers

<u>β1 stimulation</u> - ↑ contraction force + rate, AV node conduction, & renin secretion.
<u>β2 stimulation</u> - blood vessel, bronchi, GI, & GU smooth muscle relaxation.
Propranolol is nonselective, blocking β1 and β2 receptors. Other nonselective β-blockers: nadolol, timolol, pindolol. Selective β1 blockers: metoprolol, atenolol, esmolol, + acebutolol. Pindolol + acebutolol have some β agonist properties.

System	Clinical Features
CNS	• Coma and seizures (esp. with lipid soluble agents – propranolol)
Cardiac	• ↓HR, AV block (1st, 2nd or 3rd), ↑QRS, ↑ T waves, + ST changes • ↑HR with pindolol, practolol, and sotalol. ↓BP is common. • Congestive heart failure can occur.
Pulmonary	• Bronchospasm and respiratory arrest can occur.
Metabolic	• Hypoglycemia is uncommon in adults.

Treatment of β-blocker Toxicity

Option	Recommendations
Gastrointestinal decontamination	• Avoid ipecac. Aspiration & asystole are reported. • Charcoal - repeated doses, ± preceded by gastric lavage
Glucagon	• Indications: ↓HR or BP. Administer 5 mg IV then 1-5 mg/h
Atropine	• Has no effect on BP and will only ↑HR in 25%. • No HR response to 1 mg is diagnostic of β-blocker toxicity. Administer 0.5 mg IV prn (maximum of 2 mg).
Fluid/pressors	• If ↓BP does not respond to NS, administer α + β agonists (epinephrine/norepinephrine) or β agonists (dobutamine)
Other options	• Use pacemaker if no response to above. Consider dialysis if atenolol, nadolol, or acebutolol overdose. • Amrinone–consult pharmacist, specialized dosing/monitoring

Calcium Channel Blockers

System	Clinical Features
CNS	• Lethargy, slurred speech, confusion, coma, seizure, ↓respirations
Cardiac	• ↓HR, ↓BP, AV block (1st, 2nd or 3rd), sinus arrest, asystole
GI	• Nausea, vomiting, ileus, obstruction, bowel ischemia/infarction
Metabolic	• Hyperglycemia (esp. verapamil), lactic acidosis

Option	Treatment Recommendations
Gastrointestinal decontamination	• Charcoal ± preceded by gastric lavage • Avoid ipecac as aspiration, and rapid ↓mental status occurs • Whole bowel irrigation if sustained-release preparation
Calcium	• Usually ineffective at improving cardiac conduction defects • Primary indication is to reverse hypotension • Administer calcium gluconate 3 g (30 ml of 10% solution) IV over 5 minutes, repeat prn. Alternatively, administer 10 ml of calcium chloride 10% IV over 5 minutes.
Glucagon	• Indications: ↓HR or BP. Administer 5 mg IV
Atropine	• 0.5 mg IV if symptomatic↓HR (repeat X 3) – often ineffective
Fluids/pressors	• ↓BP primarily occurs from peripheral vasodilation, therefore administer fluids followed by vasoconstrictors (e.g. norepinephrine, Neo-Synephrine or high dose dopamine).
Other options	• Use pacemaker if no response to above. • High dose insulin infusion (0.1 – 1 U/kg/hour) with dextrose infusion (usually D10W-D25W) to maintain normal serum glucose levels (*J Toxicol Clin Toxicol* 1999;3:463-74.)

Carbon Monoxide

Carbon monoxide (CO) exposure can occur from fire, catabolism of heme compounds, cigarettes, pollution, ice-surfacing machines, & methylene chloride (inhaled or dermally-absorbed paint remover) degradation. CO displaces O_2 off Hb. O_2-Hb dissociation curve shifts to left. CO binds cytochrome-A, cardiac/skeletal muscle myoglobin.

FIO_2	CO half-life
room air	320 min
100% rebreather	80 min
3 ATM hyperbaric O_2	23 min

Clinical Features

CO-Hb level	Typical symptoms at given level of CO toxicity
0-10%	Usually none, ±↓exercise tolerance, ↑angina, and ↑claudication
10-20%	Frontal headache, dyspnea with exertion
20-30%	Throbbing headache, dyspnea with exertion, ↓concentration
30-40%	Severe headache, vomiting, visual changes
40-50%	Confusion, syncope on exertion, myocardial ischemia
50-60%	Collapse, seizures
> 60-70%	Coma and death
Variable	Cherry red skin, visual field defect, homonymous hemianopsia, papilledema, retinal bleed, hearing changes, pulmonary edema.

- CO poisoning may present with flu-like symptoms. Consider this diagnosis especially when multiple family members present with these complaints.
- *Delayed neuropsychiatric syndrome:* Certain patients develop permanent neurological or psychiatric abnormalities 3 days to 3 weeks after exposure. There are no reliable predictors of this syndrome, including CO-Hb levels.

Assessment of CO Intoxication

CO-Hb levels	Levels are unreliable & may be low in significant intoxication.
Anion gap	Cyanide and lactic acidosis may contribute to anion gap
Saturation gap	Calculated – directly measured arterial O_2 saturation. This gap also occurs with methemoglobin & sulfhemoglobin.
ECG	May show changes consistent with myocardial ischemia.
Cardiac markers	May be elevated from direct myocardial damage.

Treatment of CO toxicity

Criteria for Admission	Criteria for hyperbaric oxygen [1]
<ul><li>All with CO-Hb > 15-20%</li><li>Pregnancy and CO-Hb > 10%</li><li>Acidosis, ECG changes, chest pain, abnormal neurologic exam or history of unconsciousness</li><li>Persistent symptoms following 100% O_2 X 3 hours</li></ul>	<ul><li>*Absolute:* cyanide toxic, coma, un-conscious > 20 min, abnormal neurological examination, abnormal ECG, arrhythmias, CO-Hb > 25%, pH < 7.20, or neurologic symptoms after 100% O_2 X 3 h</li><li>*Relative:* pregnancy, CO-Hb > 20%.</li></ul>

1 Exact utility and indications for hyperbaric oxygen are controversial.

Clonidine

Clonidine is an α-adrenergic agonist that lowers BP, and ameliorates opiate withdrawal. Clonidine tablets (*Catapres*), in combination with chlorthalidone (*Combipres*), and transdermal patches (*Catapres*-TTS) are available. Leftover patches may contain up to 2 mg of active drug. Clonidine is rapidly absorbed from GI tract lowering BP within 30-60 min peaking at 2-4 h.

Serum half-life is 12 h (6-24 h). Clonidine lowers BP at the presynaptic α_2-agonist receptors resulting in $\downarrow$ sympathetic outflow. At high doses, it is a peripheral α-agonist + causes $\uparrow$ BP. It is also a CNS depressant.

Clinical Features of Clonidine Toxicity

CNS	• Lethargy, coma, recurrent apnea, miosis, hypotonia
Cardiac	• Sinus bradycardia, hypertension (transient), later hypotension
Other	• Hypothermia and pallor

Treatment

Monitor	• Apply cardiac monitor + pulse oximeter and observe closely for apnea. Apnea often responds to tactile stimulation.
Decontamination	• Charcoal $\pm$ gastric lavage. Avoid ipecac.
Atropine	• Indication: bradycardia. Dose: 0.5 mg IV.
Antihypertensives	• Hypertension is transient & usually no treatment is required. If needed, use short acting titratable agent (e.g. *Nipride*).
Fluids/pressors	• Treat hypotension with fluids and dopamine prn.
Naloxone	• 2 mg IV may reverse CNS but not cardiac/BP effects.

Cocaine

Cocaine is the HCl salt of the alkaloid extract of the *Erythroxylon coca* plant. It can be absorbed across all mucous membranes. It is a local anesthetic.

Route	Peak effect	Duration
Nasal	30 min	1 – 3 hr
GI	90 min	3 hr
IV/Inhaled	1 - 2 min	$\leq$ 30 min

(ester-type) that blocks the reuptake of norepinephrine, dopamine, & serotonin

Clinical Features of Cocaine Toxicity

General	• Agitation, hyperthermia, sweating, rhabdomyolysis, GI perf./ischemia
Cardiac	• A direct myocardial depressant, prolongs QT with sympathetic hyperactivity, myocardial ischemia (often with atypical clinical features & ECG findings - acutely or during withdrawal), $\uparrow$BP, $\uparrow$HR, LVH, arrhythmias, $\uparrow$platelet aggregation, accelerated atherosclerosis
CNS	• Seizures, CNS infarct or bleed, CNS abscess, vasculitis, dystonia
Lung	• Pneumothorax/mediastinum, hemorrhage, pneumonitis, ARDS

Management of Cocaine Toxicity

General	• Apply cardiac monitor, oxygen, pulse oximeter and observe closely for arrhythmia, seizures, and hyperthermia. Benzodiazepines are drug of choice for agitation, while *Haldol* is also effective (without ↑ cocaine seizure threshold)
Hyperthermia & Rhabdomyolysis	• Benzodiazepines to reduce agitation and muscle activity. Cool with mist and fan. Continuous rectal probe temperature. Check serum CK/CO_2. Administer IV fluids & bicarbonate to prevent renal failure (page 57).
GI decontaminate	• *Body stuffers* – charcoal & monitor for perforation/ischemia • *Body packer* – Xray and whole bowel irrigation. If rupture, consider laparotomy to remove cocaine
Cardiovascular (*Arrhythmias & Hypertension*)	• Administer benzodiazepines for ↑BP, ↑HR. Treat according to standard ACLS protocols: Avoid β blockade (unopposed alpha). Use caution with labetalol (β > α block ± ↑ seizures). Use sodium nitroprusside (*Nipride*) or phentolamine for severe HTN. • <u>Wide complex tachycardia</u> is due to quinidine-like effect. Administer bicarbonate and cardiovert. Avoid β blockers.
Cardiovascular (*Chest pain*)	• Administer benzodiazepines, aspirin, and IV NTG. Alternately, phentolamine IV may reverse coronary vasoconstriction. PTCA is preferred over thrombolytics as CNS bleed/vasculitis/HTN ↑ risk of CNS bleed.
Neurologic	• Treat status epilepticus with benzodiazepines. Barbiturates are 2nd line while phenytoin is not useful. Exclude coexisting pathology (CT, glucose, electrolytes, infection).

Digoxin

Natural sources: foxglove, oleander, lily of the valley, and the skin of toads. Therapeutic range - 0.6-1.2 ng/ml. Severe poisoning may not demonstrate ↑levels.

Clinical Features – Acute Toxicity

Digoxin level	Usually markedly elevated (obtain > 6 hours after ingestion)
GI and CNS	Nausea, vomiting, diarrhea, headache, confusion, coma
Cardiac	Supraventricular tachycardia, AV blocks, bradyarrhythmias
Metabolic	Hyperkalemia from inhibition of the Na^+/K^+ ATP pump

Clinical Features – Chronic Toxicity

Digoxin level	May be normal
History	URI symptoms, on diuretics, renal insufficiency, yellow-green halos
Cardiac	Ventricular arrhythmias are more common than with acute toxicity
Metabolic	Potassium low or normal, magnesium is often low

Treatment of Digoxin Toxicity	
• Multi-dose charcoal ± lavage.	• ↑K⁺: page 47. Do not use calcium.
• Atropine 0.5 mg for ↓HR	• Avoid cardioversion if possible (pre-
• Ventricular arrhythmia: lidocaine 1	disposes to ventricular fibrillation).
mg/kg IV ± MgSO₄ 20 mg/kg IV	• Digoxin Fab fragments (*Digibind*)

Indications for Digibind	Total body load digoxin - TBLD estimates
• Ventricular arrhythmias	TBLD (total body load of digoxin) in milligrams =
• Symptomatic bradyarrhy-	• [digoxin level[1] (ng/ml) x weight (kg)] ÷ 100
thmias unresponsive to Rx	• (Acute ingestion) - total mg ingested if digoxin
• Ingestion of > 0.1 mg/kg	capsules or elixir is ingested
• Digoxin level of > 5 ng/ml	• (Acute ingestion) - total mg ingested X 0.8 if
• Consider if K⁺ >5-5.5 mEq/l	digoxin tables (due to 80% bioavailability)

[1] *Chronic ingestions* may have normal to mildly elevated digoxin levels.

Digibind Dosing
• Number of vials to administer = TBLD in mg divided by 0.5 (mg/vial)
• If ingested quantity unknown consider empiric administration of 10 vials
• One 40 mg *Digibind* vial can bind 0.5 mg of digoxin if amount ingested known
• Dilute *Digibind* to 10 mg/ml & administer IV over 30 min. Consider using 0.22 micron filter for infusion. Serum levels are useless after use assay measures bound + unbound digoxin. Once bound, digoxin-Fab complex is renally excreted.

Flunitrazepam - *Rohypnol "Roofies"*

Rohypnol is a benzodiazepine marketed outside the US for insomnia, sedation, & pre-anesthesia. It is 10 X as potent as diazepam. It potentiates and prolongs the effects of heroin, methadone, & alcohol and attenuates the withdrawal of cocaine. It produces disinhibition and amnesia and has been used as a "date rape" drug.

Onset/duration	• Maximal absorption is 0.5-1.5 hr with T½ of nearly 12 hours.
Major clinical effects	• CNS - sedation, incoordination, hallucinations. Paradoxical excitement, esp. with alcohol use. ↓DTRs, mid to small pupils.
	• CV-Pulm - Respiratory depression, hypotension, aspiration
Management	• NOT routinely detected in urine benzodiazepine screen
	• Lavage if < 1 hr from ingestion, otherwise administer charcoal
	• Protect airway and apply cardiac monitor, pulse oximeter
	• Admit if lethargic or unstable after 2-4 hr of observation.

Gamma Hydroxybutyric acid (GHB)

Gamma hydroxybutyric acid (GHB) has been promoted as a steroid alternative, a weight control agent, and as a narcolepsy treatment.

Onset/duration	• Onset of symptoms is ~ 15 minutes, with spont. resolution from 2 to > 48 hours (depending on dose & co-ingestant).
Major clinical effects	• <u>CNS</u> Acts synergistically with ethanol to produce CNS and respiratory depression. At high serum levels patients are unresponsive to noxious stimuli and lose pharyngeal/laryngeal reflexes. Seizures, clonic arm/leg/face movements, vomiting, amnesia,↓DTRs & vertigo occur. Nystagmus and ataxia occur. • CV-Pulm – ↓ HR, Irregular or ↓ respirations, ↓ BP.
Management	• Protect airway and apply cardiac monitor, pulse oximeter • Treat symptomatically (e.g. use atropine for persistent ↓ HR). • Exclude coingestant or alternate diagnosis (e.g. CNS trauma) • Admit if symptoms do not resolve after 6 hours of observation.

Hallucinogens

Common hallucinogens include LSD (lysergic acid diethylamide), mescaline (peyote plant), psilocybin (mushrooms – esp. from cow pastures), morning glory seeds (similar to LSD), nutmeg and toads (skin contains hallucinogenic *bufotoxins*).

Clinical Features of Hallucinogen Toxicity	
General	• Onset of symptoms is generally 30-60 minutes with 4-8 hr duration. • Sympathetic stimulation(↑pupils, diaphoresis, piloerection) • Hyperthermia, neuroleptic malignant syndrome, rhabdomyolysis (esp. if patient is restrained)
CNS	• Panic attacks with hallucinations that are often cross-sensory (tasting colors/seeing sounds), illusions, misperceptions. Seizures and coma are less common. ↑DTRs
Cardiac	• ↑ HR often with normal or mild ↑ BP.
GI	• Vomiting & diarrhea are more common with mescaline, psilocybin
Treatment	
Monitor	• Apply cardiac monitor + pulse oximeter and observe closely for seizures, agitation, hyperthermia, rhabdomyolysis
Decontamination	• Charcoal ± lavage are useful for peyote or psilocybin, but not LSD as it is too rapidly absorbed. Avoid ipecac.
Agitation	• Verbal reassurance may be useful. Benzodiazepines followed by haloperidol may be useful if severe agitation.

Lithium

Li absorption leads to peak serum levels 0.5 – 3 hr post ingestion. Significant delayed absorption/symptom onset may occur up to 72 hr later. Therapeutic serum concentrations (acute mania = 0.6-1.2 mEq/L, maintenance 0.5 – 0.8 mEq/L).

Clinical Features of Toxicity Based on Serum Levels	
Lithium level	**Clinical Features[1]**
< 1.2 mEq/L	Fine tremor, dry mouth, thirst, polyuria, nausea (not toxic signs)
1.2-2.0	Vomiting and diarrhea
2.0-2.5	Blurred vision, muscle weakness/fasciculations, dizziness, vertigo, ataxia, confusion, slurred speech, ↑ DTRs, transient scotomas
2.5-3.0	Myoclonic twitches, choreoathetoid movements, incontinence, stupor, ECG: flat/inverted T's, U wave, SA/AV block, prolonged QT.
3.0-4.0	Seizures, cardiac arrhythmias (ventricular tachycardia, PVCs, Vfib)
≥ 4.0	Hypotension, peripheral vascular collapse

Lithium may cause diabetes insipidus (↑ Na^+), ↓ anion gap, ↑ K^+ (displacement of K^+ by intracellular Li), ECG changes similar to ↓ K^+ and hypothyroidism.

[1]Serum levels do not always correlate with features, toxicity can occur with normal levels (esp. if acute on chronic ingestion).

Treatment	
Monitor	• Apply cardiac monitor, pulse oximeter, obtain ECG, serum electrolytes & observe for neurologic or cardiac deterioration • Obtain serum Li 2 h post acute and 6-12 post chronic ingestion. Repeat Li levels q 4 h until a peak is reached.
Decontamination	• Gastric lavage if recent ingestion, charcoal is ineffective • Sodium polystyrene sulfonate (*Kayexalate*) 1g/kg PO or PR • Whole bowel irrigation (esp. if sustained release) – pg 149
Fluids & Electrolytes	• Restore fluid, electrolyte deficits (NS administration supplies Na^+ ions which may increase renal Li excretion). • Controversy exists regarding use of $NaHCO_3$, acetazolamide and osmotic diuretics. Contact poison center for direction.
Indications for Hemodialysis	• <u>Signs of severe poisoning</u> (e.g. seizures, altered mental status, ventricular arrhythmias) • Decreasing urine output or renal failure • Lithium level ≥ 4.0 mEq/L regardless of symptoms • Repeat dialysis is often needed 6-12 h later due to slow distribution. Check levels q 4h post dialysis X 12-24 h

Mushrooms

Treat all toxic mushroom ingestions with IV fluids and GI decontamination. Specific antidotes are useful for certain mushrooms as discussed below. Toxic mushrooms Groups I, II, and VIII (cyclopeptides, monomethylhydrazines, and orellines) cause delayed symptom onset (> 6h from ingestion). Nontoxic ingestions generally cause symptoms < 6 hours after ingestion.

Phases of cyclopeptide mushroom toxicity	Phase	Time	Features
	0	0-6h	asymptomatic latent phase (may last 24h)
	1	6-12h	gastrointestinal phase: vomiting, diarrhea
	2	12-24h	symptoms ↓, ↑liver function tests
	3	>24h	liver failure, shock, renal failure

Clinical Features, Onset, and Treatment of Mushroom Toxicity

Group	Toxin	Onset	Symptoms	Treatment
I Cyclo-peptides	cyclopeptides amatoxins phallatoxins virotoxins	6-10h	See Table above	Multi-dose charcoal, IV NS, ± (penicillin G, cimetidine, thioctic acid, silymarin/silibinin)
II MMH	monomethyl-hydrazine (MMH)	6-10h	CNS-seizures abdominal pain hepatorenal failure	Pyridoxine 25 mg/kg IV or greater, Methylene blue for methemoglobinemia
III Muscarine	muscarine	½ - 2h	Cholinergic	Atropine if ↓ HR
VI Coprine	coprine	½ - 2h	Disulfiram reaction (↑HR, flushed, vomit)	IV fluids
V Ibotenic acid and muscimol	ibotenic acid, muscimol	½ - 2h	GABA effects: (seizures, hal-lucinations), Anticholinergic	Benzodiazepines
VI Psilocybin	psilocybin psilocin	½ - 1h	Hallucinations (~LSD)	Benzodiazepines
VII GI toxins	multiple	½ - 3h	Pain, vomiting, diarrhea	IV fluids
VIII Orellines	orelline, orellanine	24 - 36h	Renal failure, vomiting	Supportive care, ± dialysis

Neuroleptics

Side effects of neuroleptics include
(1) anti-adrenergic - ↓BP, ↑ HR
(2) anticholinergic - ↑ temp, dry,
urine retention, ↑pupils (phenothiazines may cause ↓pupils), CNS
and respiratory depression
(3) anti-dopaminergic – dystonia,
akithisia, motor disorders,
(4) quinidine effect on heart (↑QT,
↑PR, torsades). Low potency drugs
Thorazine, Serentil have more anti-cholinergic/anti-adrenergic effect,
while ↑ potency butyrophenones &
thioxanthenes have more antidopa-mine effects. Thioridazine & mesoridazine have most quinidine-like cardiac effect.

Class	Example Drugs
Butyrophenone	droperidol *Inapsine*
	haloperidol *Haldol*
Dibenzazepine	loxapine *Loxitane*
Dihydroindolone	molindone *Moban*
Phenothiazines	chlorpromazine *Thorazine*
	fluphenazine *Prolixin*
	mesoridazine *Serentil*
	perphenazine *Trilafon*
	prochlorperazine *Compazine*
	promethazine *Phenergan*
	thioridazine *Mellaril*
	trifluoperazine *Stelazine*
Thioxanthenes	thiothixene *Navane*

Treatment	
Monitor	• Apply cardiac monitor + pulse oximeter and obtain ECG.
GI decontaminate	• Charcoal 1g/kg PO, consider lavage 1st
Hypotension	• NS IV, if unresponsive use α agonist (e.g. norepinephrine)
Ventricular Arrhythmias	• NaHCO$_3$ 1 mEq/kg IV, may repeat.
	• Lidocaine or Amiodarone per protocol – page 207
	• Magnesium 2-4 g IV over 15 min (if no renal insufficiency)
	• Avoid Class IA anti-arrhythmics (e.g. procainamide)
Medically admit	• All who are symptomatic or become symptomatic over 6 h (e.g. ↓BP, altered mental status, arrhythmia, ECG changes)
	• All thioridazine or mesoridazine ingestions (delayed VF/VT)

Phencyclidine (PCP)

Three stages of intoxication are (1) acute organic brain syndrome with violent behavior (2) progressive stupor with intact pain response, and (3) deep coma.

Clinical features: Mixed adrenergic (↑BP,↑HR, hyperthermia, mydriasis), and cholinergic (miosis, sweating, wheezing, salivation) features. Nystagmus (any direction), with blank open-eyed stare and roving gave. Rhabdomyolysis, CNS bleed, stridor, DIC, respiratory depression, and seizures occur.

Management: Sedate (benzodiazepines ± haloperidol) and restraint patient for protection. Monitor neurologic, cardiac, and pulmonary status. Exclude life threats (e.g. hyperthermia, rhabdomyolysis). Consider repeat doses of charcoal.

Insecticides - Organophosphates and Carbamates

Organophosphates irreversibly bind and inhibit cholinesterases at CNS receptors, post-ganglionic parasympathetic nerves (muscarinic effects), and autonomic ganglia and skeletal myoneural junctions (nicotinic effects). Carbamates reversibly bind cholinesterases and are less toxic than organophosphates.

	Clinical Features of Insecticide Toxicity
Onset of symptoms	• Usually < 24h after exposure. Lipid-soluble organophosphates (e.g. fenthion) may take days to cause symptoms & last months
CNS	• Cholinergic excess: delirium, confusion, seizures, respiratory depression. Carbamates have less central effects.
Muscarinic	• SLUDGE (salivation, lacrimation, urination, defecation, GI upset, emesis), miosis, bronchoconstriction, bradycardia.
Nicotinic	• Fasciculations, muscle weakness, sympathetic ganglia stimulation (hypertension, tachycardia, pallor, rarely mydriasis)
	Diagnostic Studies in Insecticide Poisoning
Labs	• ↑glucose,↑K⁺,↑WBC,↑amylase, glycosuria, proteinuria
ECG	• Early - ↑ in sympathetic tone (tachycardia) • Later - extreme parasympathetic tone (sinus bradycardia, AV block, and ↑QT).
Serum *(pseudo)* RBC *(plasma)* Cholinesterase	• Serum levels are more sensitive but less specific than RBC • Plasma levels return to normal before RBC levels • Mild cases: levels are < 50% of normal • Severe cases: levels are < 10% of normal
	Treatment
General	• Support airway, breathing and blood pressure. Respiratory depression is the most common cause of death. • Medical personnel should gown and glove if dermal exposure. • Wash toxin off patient if dermal exposure. • Administer charcoal if oral ingestion.
Atropine	• Competitively blocks acetylcholine at muscarinic (not nicotinic) receptors. Atropine may reverse CNS effects. • <u>Dose</u>: 1-2 mg (or >) q 5 min. Mix 50 mg in 500 ml NS and titrate • <u>Goal</u>: titrate to mild anticholinergic signs (dry mouth, secretions) and not to pupil size or heart rate. • Treatment failure is due to not using enough atropine.
Pralidoxime (2-PAM)	• Reverses nicotinic & central effects, not carbamate toxicity. • <u>Dose</u>: 1 g IV over 15 minutes. May repeat in 1 hour then q3-8 hours prn. Onset of effect is 10-40 minutes after administration.
Atrovent	• Ipratropium bromide 0.5 mg nebulized may dry secretions.

Salicylates

Methylsalicylate (oil of wintergreen) is the most toxic form. Absorption generally is within 1h of ingestion (delays $\geq$ 6h occur with enteric-coated and viscous preparations. At toxic levels, salicylates are renally metabolized. Alkaline urine promotes excretion. At different acidosis/alkalosis states, measurable salicylate levels change, therefore measure arterial pH at same time as drug level.

Ingestion	Severity	Signs and Symptoms
<150 mg/kg	mild	vomiting, tinnitus, and hyperpnea
150-300 mg/kg	moderate	vomiting, hyperpnea, diaphoresis, and tinnitus
>300 mg/kg	severe	acidosis, altered mental status, seizures, & shock

Clinical Features of Salicylate Toxicity

Direct	• Irritation of GI tract with reports of perforation
Metabolic	• Early: respiratory alkalosis from respiratory center stimulation
	• Later: metabolic acidosis - uncoupled oxidative phosphorylation
	• Hypokalemia, ↑or↓ glucose, ketonuria, and either ↑or↓ Na+
CNS	• Early: tinnitus, deafness, agitation, hyperactivity,
	• Later: confusion, lethargy, coma, seizure, CNS edema (esp. < 4y)
GI	• Vomiting, gastritis, pylorospasm, ↑ liver enzymes, perforation
Pulmonary	• Noncardiac pulmonary edema (esp. with chronic toxicity)

Indicators of Salicylate Toxicity

Clinical	• Features listed above are associated with toxicity
Ingestion	• Ingestion of > 150 mg/kg may be associated with toxicity
Ferric chloride	• Mix 2 drops $FeCl_3$+ 1 ml urine. Purple = salicylate ingestion
Phenstix	• Dipstick test for urine. Brown indicates salicylate or pheno-thiazine ingestion (not toxicity). Adding 1 drop 20N H_2SO_4 bleaches out color for phenothiazines but not salicylates.
Salicylate Levels	• A level > 30 mg/dl drawn $\geq$ 6h after ingestion is toxic. Clinical findings are more important than serum levels.
	• Follow serial levels (q2-3h) until downward trend established
	• Arterial pH must be measured at same time, as acidemia increases CNS penetration and toxicity at lower levels.
	• *Done nomogram has been proven unreliable*
Nontoxic Ingestion	• If none of the following are present, acute toxicity is unlikely (1) < 150 mg/kg ingested, (2) absent clinical features (3) level < 30 mg/dl obtained $\geq$ 6h after ingestion (unless enteric coated preparation, viscous preparation, or chronic ingestion)

Treatment of Acute Salicylate Toxicity	
General	• Treat dehydration, electrolyte abnormalities. CSF hypoglycemia occurs with normal serum glucose – add D_5 or D_{10} to all fluids.
Decontaminate	• Multi-dose charcoal, Whole bowel irrigation (if enteric coated)
Alkalinization	• Add 100 mEq $NaHCO_3$ to 1 L D_5NS (20-40 mEq/L K^+ if no renal failure). Infuse at 200 ml/hour. *Goal* – urine pH > 7.5
Hemodialysis	• *Indications*: renal failure, noncardiogenic pulmonary edema, CHF, persistent CNS disturbances, ↓BP, unable to correct acid-base or electrolyte imbalance, salicylate level > 100 mg/dl

Chronic Salicylate Toxicity	
Presentation	• Older, chronic salicylates, altered CNS, non-cardiogenic pulmonary edema. ± Misdiagnosed as infectious/neuro disease.
Drug levels	• Salicylate levels are often normal to therapeutic.
Treatment	• Supportive measures and urinary alkalinization. Dialyze if acidosis, confusion, or pulmonary edema even if level normal.

Selective Serotonin Reuptake Inhibitors & Non-Tricyclic antidepressants

Selective serotonin reuptake inhibitors (SSRIs)	SSRIs
OD is relatively benign (morbidity related to co-ingestants) Most common symptoms: ↑ HR, tremor, vomiting, and drowsiness. ECG: ↑ HR, non-specific ST-T changes. Seizures and cardiotoxicity (wide QRS/QTc) can occur at high levels (esp. fluoxetine). ↓ HR is seen with fluvoxamine at high or low doses. *Treatment*: (1) exclude coingestants (2) observe for 6 hours (3) Charcoal 1g/kg (4) Sodium bicarbonate IV is useful if wide QRS tachycardia, (5) Observe for *Serotonin Syndrome* – see page 164.	citalopram (*Celexa*) escitalopram (*Lexapro*) fluoxetine (*Prozac*) fluvoxamine (*Luvox*) paroxetine (*Paxil*) sertraline (*Zoloft*)
MAOI OD may have onset up 12 h later. Excess α+β adrenergic symptoms: Headache, tremor, ↑BP,↑DTR rigidity, chest pain, ↑temp. Later ↓BP, ↓HR, seizures *Treatment:* (1) Nipride or phentolamine for ↑ BP [No β blockers] (2) NS + Norepi. for ↓ BP (3) Charcoal (4) benzodiazepines (5) treat rhabdomyolysis, ↑ temp (6) Admit all intentional OD & all ingestions > 2 mg/kg	**Monoamine oxidase inhibitors (MAOIs)** isocarboxazid (*Marplan*) phenylzine (*Nardil*) selegiline (*Eldepryl*) tranylcypromine (*Parnate*)

Other Non-Tricyclic antidepressants

Serotonin, Norepinephrine reuptake inhibitors – Venlafaxine (*Effexor*) – OD causes ↑ HR and ↓ level of consciousness, brief and limited seizures, mild hypotension. Treat with supportive care, benzodiazepines if seizures, saline and vasopressors for hypotension.

Norepinephrine & Dopamine reuptake inhibitor – bupropion (*Wellbutrin*). OD causes lethargy (41%), tremors (24%), and seizures (21%). Mean onset of seizures was 3.7 hours and responds to benzodiazepines, and phenytoin. Single case report of prolonged QRS/QTc. Treat supportively.

Noradrenergic & Serotoninergic antidepressants – mirtazapine (*Remeron*) inhibits presynaptic $\alpha 2$ receptors increasing serotonin and norepinephrine transmission. Serotonin-2 and 3 receptors are blocked diminishing anxiety and GI side effects. OD is rare with sedation and drowsiness requiring rare intubation. No cardiac conduction effects or seizures have been noted to date.

Serotonin-2 receptor antagonists – nefazodone (*Serzone*) and trazodone (*Desyrel*) block serotonin reuptake and inhibit serotonin-2 receptors. Nefazodone also blocks norepinephrine reuptake and had minimal $\alpha 1$ receptor antagonism. Both (esp. trazodone) cause sedation, lightheadedness, GI upset, headaches. Trazodone has been associated with nonsustained ventricular tachycardia and other dysrhythmias. Treatment for OD of either agent is supportive.

Serotonin Syndrome –hyperserotoninergic cluster: encephalopathy (40%), ↑DTRs rigid muscles (rhabdomyolysis), vomit & autonomic instability (↑temp 50%, sweat). *Select causes:* Drug interactions between SSRIs, TCAs, MAOIs, meperidine, codeine, and dextromethorphan. Patients with serotonin syndrome have more GI features, myoclonus, ↑DTR compared to neuroleptic malignant syndrome.
Treatment: Stop drug, manage complications (hyperthermia/rhabdomyolysis), benzodiazepines, ± cyproheptadine (serotonin antagonist) 4-8 mg PO q 8 h.

Sympathomimetics (Amphetamines & Derivatives)

Effects of amphetamines are (1) <u>sympathomimetic</u> - α & β adrenergic - mydriasis, ↑HR, ↑BP, ↑temp., arrhythmias, MI, rhabdomyolysis, psychosis, CNS bleed, ↑sweat, seizures (2) <u>dopaminergic</u> - restless, anorexia, hyperactive, movement disorders, paranoia (3) <u>serotonergic</u> – mood, impulse control, serotonin syndrome

Ice/crank (crystal methamphetamine) 1 of most commonly synthesized illicit drugs. Onset is minutes, lasts 2-24 h. **MDMA – Ecstasy** – popular at "raves" and consumed orally. Low dose - euphoria, mild sympathomimetic symptoms last ~ 4-6 h. Potent serotonin releaser (no impulse control). High dose - effects (1-3) above in addition to hyponatremia.

Treatment (1) supportive care, cardiopulmonary & neuro monitoring, (2) anticipate complications, (3) benzodiazepines for agitation, (4) labetalol or Nipride– 1st line for ↑ BP (5) If ↓ BP, dopamine or norepinephrine (6) charcoal if oral ingestion, (7) treat MI, dysrhythmias, hyperthermia and rhabdomyolysis in standard fashion.

Theophylline

Clinical Features	
Cardiovascular	• Tachycardia, atrial and ventricular dysrhythmias
Neurological	• Agitation, tremors, seizures
Metabolic	• ↑Glucose, ↑catecholamines, ↓potassium
Gastrointestinal	• Vomiting

Treatment	
General	• Monitor for seizures, arrhythmias. Correct dehydration, hypoxia, and electrolyte imbalances.
Charcoal	• Administer 1g/kg q2-4h. Repeat doses q4h.
Arrhythmias	• β-blockade is preferred for tachyarrhythmias. Do not use verapamil. It inhibits theophylline metabolism.
Seizures	• Use benzodiazepines and barbiturates (not phenytoin).
Hemoperfusion Indications	• (1) seizures, (2) poorly responsive arrhythmias, (3) level > 100 µg/ml in acute overdose > 60 µg/ml in chronic overdose

TOXIC ALCOHOLS: Ethanol

Ethanol (EtOH) contributes 22 mOsm/L for every 100mg/dl to serum osmolality. Mean elimination of ethanol is 20 mg/dl/h (range 16-25) *Am J Emerg Med* 1995; 276.

Clinical Features	
CNS	• Euphoria, disinhibition, sedation, Wernicke-Korsakoff syndrome
Cardiac	• ↑HR, ↓BP, atrial (esp. atrial fibrillation) & ventricular arrhythmias
Respiratory	• Aspiration, bradypnea
GI	• Vomiting, bleeding, ulcer, gastritis, hepatitis, pancreatitis
Metabolic	• ↑or↓temperature, ↓glucose, ↓Mg, ketoacidosis

Alcoholic Ketoacidosis

	Laboratory values
Due to an ethanol binge in patient who has a decreased caloric intake. Keto-acids, β-hydroxybutyric acid (βHB) and acetoacetate (AcA) accumulate in blood.	• Anion gap metabolic acidosis • Positive Nitroprusside test (serum and urine) detecting acetoacetate • Low, normal or mildly ↑glucose
Clinical Features	
• Vomiting, anorexia, abdominal pain • Hypothermia, dehydration, • ↑HR,↓BP, dehydration,↓urination • Recently terminated alcoholic binge • Poor caloric intake X 24-72 hours	*Management* • Rehydration (D₅NS or D₅½NS) • Thiamine 100 mg before glucose • Correct electrolyte disturbances • Do not administer bicarbonate

Ethylene Glycol

Ethylene glycol is found in coolants (e.g. automobile anti-freeze), preservatives, lacquers, cosmetics, polishes, and detergents.

Timing	Clinical Features
1-12 hours	• **Early**: inebriation, ataxia, slurring without ethanol on breath • **Later**: coma, seizures, and death
12-24 hours	• Cardiac deterioration occurs during this phase • **Early**: tachycardia, hypertension, tachypnea • **Later**: congestive heart failure, ARDS, and cardiovascular collapse • Myositis occasionally occurs during this phase
24-72 hours	• Nephrotoxicity with calcium oxalate crystal precipitation leading to flank pain, renal failure, and hypocalcemia

Diagnosis	Treatment
• Anion gap acidosis • Osmol gap[2] (measured – calculated osmol) > 10 mOsm/L (page 7) • Hypocalcemia (ECG - ↑QT interval) • Calcium oxalate crystals in urine • ↑BUN and creatinine • Serum ethylene glycol level > 20 mg/dl is toxic • Serious toxicity has been reported in the <u>absence</u> of anion gap/crystalluria	• Gastric lavage (charcoal is ineffective) • NaHCO₃ 50 mEq IV to keep pH ~7.40 • Ca⁺² gluconate 10%, 10-20 ml IV if ↓Ca⁺², MgSO₄ 2g IV over 15-30 min • Pyridoxine/thiamine, each 100 mg IV • Fomepizole[1] (*Antizol*) – 15 mg/kg IV, + 10 mg/kg q12h X 4 doses, then ↑ to 15 mg/kg IV q12h until level < 20mg/dl • Dialysis if (1) oliguria/anuria, (2) severe acidosis, or (3) level > 50 mg/dl (> 20 mg/dl if fomepizole not used)

[1] Administer slow IV over 15 min. If unavailable, load IV ethanol (see Methanol).
[2] Osmol gap may be normal in significant toxicity.

Isopropanol

Isopropanol sources: rubbing alcohol, skin and hair products, jewelry cleaners, paint thinners, and antifreeze. Toxicity occurs after ingestion, inhalation, or dermal exposure (e.g. sponge bath).

Clinical Features	Diagnosis
• Onset of symptoms within 1 hour	• Osmol gap (see page 7)
• Inebriation, CNS depression, coma	• Acetonemia (ketonemia), acetonuria
• Hypotension - peripheral vasodilation	• Normal or mild ↓ pH (no anion gap)
• Abdominal pain, vomiting, ↓glucose	• Isopropanol > 50 mg/dl – mild
• Hemorrhagic gastritis, renal failure	intoxication, > 150 mg/dl – severe
• Hemolysis, rhabdomyolysis	• ↓ or ↔ glucose, ↑BUN & creatinine

Treatment
• Gastric lavage and charcoal are generally ineffective
• Supportive care (maintaining BP and respirations) is all that is required.
• Consider hemodialysis if (1) hypotension refractory to conventional therapy or (2) predicted peak level > 400 mg/dl. Dialysis rarely required.

Methanol

Methyl alcohol sources: wood alcohol, solvents, paint removers, shellacs, windshield washing fluids, and antifreeze. Toxicity is from formaldehyde/formic acid. Death has been reported after ingestion of 15 ml of 40% solution.

Clinical Features		Treatment
0-12 hours	• Inebriation, drowsiness • Asymptomatic period	• Gastric lavage/charcoal are ineffective • $NaHCO_3$ 50 mEq IV to keep pH > 7.35
12-36 hours	• Vomiting, hyperventilation • Abdominal pain, pancreatitis • Visual blurring, blindness with mydriasis & papilledema • CNS depression	• Folate 50 mg IV q 4 hours • Fomepizole (*Antizol*) – (see ethylene glycol dosing) • Ethanol (10%) in D_5W – (1) IV loading dose 10 ml/kg over 1-2 h (2) then 100
Diagnostic Studies		mg/kg/h (3) ↑ dose 50% if chronic alcohol use, (4) Goal: ethanol level: 100-150 mg/dl

• Osmol gap[1] may occur before anion gap acidosis (see page 7)
• Anion gap and lactic acidosis
• Hemoconcentration, hyperglycemia
• Methanol levels > 20 mg/dl are toxic
  (1) CNS symptoms occur > 20 mg/dl
  (2) Visual symptoms occur > 50 mg/dl
		• Dialyze if (1) visual symptoms, (2) CNS depression, (3) level > 50 mg/dl, (4) severe metabolic acidosis, or (5) history of ingestion of > 30 ml.
		• Stop dialysis and ethanol when methanol levels fall to < 20 mg/dl.

[1] Osmol gap may be normal in significant toxicity.

Tricyclic Antidepressants (TCA)

Clinical features are due to:	ECG findings in TCA overdose
• α adrenergic blockade ($\downarrow$BP), • Anti-cholinergic effects (altered mental status, seizures, $\uparrow$HR, mydriasis), • Inhibition of norepinephrine uptake (increasing catecholamines) • Na^+ channel block (causing quinidine like depressive effect on the heart)	• Sinus tachycardia • $\uparrow$QRS > 100 ms[1], $\uparrow$PR interval, $\uparrow$QT interval, BBB[2] (esp. right BBB) • Right axis deviation of the terminal 40 ms of the QRS > 120 degrees (prominent terminal R in AVR) • AV conduction blocks (all degrees) • Ventricular fibrillation or tachycardia

[1]ms – milliseconds; [2]bundle branch block

Treatment of TCA Toxicity

General	• Apply cardiac monitor, obtain baseline ECG to assess QRS width and QT interval
Decontamination	• Administer charcoal 1 g/kg PO or NG q2-4h. • Consider gastric lavage as anticholinergic effects may slow gastric emptying. • Ensure patent airway & gag reflex prior to decontamination. • Avoid ipecac, as patients may have rapid mental status decline or develop seizures.
$NaHCO_3$	• <u>Indications</u>: (1) acidosis, (2) QRS width > 100 milliseconds, (3) ventricular arrhythmias, or (4) hypotension. • Alkalinization enhances TCA protein binding and reverses Na^+ channel blockade and toxic cardiac manifestations. • <u>Dose</u>: 1-2 mEq/kg IV. May repeat. • <u>Goal</u>: Arterial pH of 7.50-7.55. • $NaHCO_3$ is ineffective for CNS side effects (e.g. seizures).
Fluids/pressors	• Administer 1-2 L NS for hypotension. Repeat 1-2 X. • If fluids are ineffective administer phenylephrine or norepinephrine (not dopamine) due to α-agonist effects.
Anti-seizure medications	• Use lorazepam followed by phenobarbital if seizure occurs. • Phenytoin is ineffective in TCA-induced seizures.
$MgSO_4$	• 25 mg/kg IV (over 15 min) may be useful for cardiac toxicity.
Disposition	*Transfer to a psychiatric facility if all of the following are present:* • no major evidence of toxicity during 6h ED observation • active bowel sounds and $\geq$ 2 charcoal doses are given • there is no evidence of toxic coingestant.

Initial Approach to Trauma Assessment and Management

PRIMARY SURVEY	
Assess **Airway** (*immobilize Cspine*)	• If poor or no air movement, perform jaw thrust or insert oral or nasal airway. • Intubate if Glasgow coma scale ≤ 8, poor response to above, severe shock, flail chest or need to hyperventilate. • Cricothyrotomy or laryngeal mask airway if unsuccessful
Assess **Breathing**	• Examine neck and thorax to detect deviated trachea, flail chest, sucking chest wound and breath sounds. • Needle chest for tension pneumothorax, apply occlusive dressing to 3 sides of sucking chest wound, reposition ET tube, or insert chest tubes (36-38 Fr) if needed. • Administer O_2, apply pulse oximeter, measure ET CO_2.
Assess **Circulation**	• Apply pressure to external bleeding sites, establish 2 large peripheral IV lines, obtain blood for basic labs and type and crossmatch, administer 2L NS IV prn. • Check pulses, listen for heart sounds, observe neck veins, assess cardiac rhythm & treat cardiac tamponade. • Apply cardiac monitor, obtain BP, HR (pulse quality)
Assess **Disability** (*neurologic status*)	• Measure Glasgow Coma Scale or assess if • **A**lert, or respond to **V**erbal, **P**ainful, **U**nresponsive to pain • Pupil assessment - size, and reactivity
Patient **Exposure**	• Completely undress patient (but keep warm).
RESUSCITATION (Perform simultaneously during primary survey)	
Reassess ABCD's	• Reassess ABCs if patient deteriorates. Address abnormality as identified, place chest tube if needed. • Emergent thoracotomy if > 1.2-1.5 L of blood from initial chest tube, > 100-200 ml/h after 1st h, or persistent ↓ BP • Administer 2nd 2L NS bolus, then blood prn. • Place NG tube + Foley catheter (unless contraindicated).
SECONDARY SURVEY	
History	• Obtain *AMPLE* history (*A*llergies, *M*edications, *P*ast History, *L*ast meal, and *E*vents leading up to injury)
Physical exam	• Perform head to toe examination (including rectal/back).
Xrays	• Obtain cervical spine, chest, pelvic films, CT scans etc.
Address injuries	• Reduce/splint fractures, call consultants as soon as needed, administer analgesics, tetanus, + antibiotics prn.
Disposition	• Initiate transfer, admit, or ready OR. Document all findings, xrays, labs, consultants, and talk to family.

Trauma Score

Respiratory rate	Systolic BP	GCS[1]	Respiratory effort
2. ≥ 36/min	4. ≥ 90mmHg	5. GCS 14-15	1. Normal
3. 25-35/min	3. 70-89 mm Hg	4. GCS 11-13	0. Shallow
4. 10-24/min	2. 50-69 mm Hg	3. GCS 8-10	0. Retractive
1. 0-9/min	1. 0-49 mm Hg	2. GCS 5-7	**Capillary refill**
0. None	0. No pulse	1. GCS 3-4	2. Normal

≤ 12 total points needs trauma center, > 14 < 1% mortality, 13-14 (1-2% risk), 11-12 (2.5% risk), ≤10 (> 10% risk). · 1. Delayed · 0. None

[1]GCS – Glasgow coma score   *Ann Emerg Med 1988; 895.*

Glasgow Coma Scale*

Eye opening	Best verbal	Best motor
4. spontaneous	5. oriented, converses	6. obeys 5. localize pain
3. to verbal command	4. disoriented, converses	4. withdrawal
2. to pain	3. inappropriate words	3. abnormal flexion/decorticate
1. no response	2. incomprehensible	2. extension/decerebrate
	1. no response	1. no response

*Total score indicates mild (13-15), moderate (9-12), or severe (≤ 8) head injury.

American College of Surgeons' Classification of Shock

Class	Blood Volume Lost	Signs and Symptoms
I	< 15% (< 750 ml if 70 kg)	Normal HR, normal vitals, few symptoms
II	15-30% (750-1500 ml)	HR > 100, ↓ pulse pressure, anxiety, urine output - 20-30 ml/h, capillary refill > 2 sec, RR 20-30
III	30-40% (1500-2000 ml)	HR > 120, ↓ BP, RR 30-40, confused, urine output - 5-15 ml/h, capillary refill > 2 sec.
IV	> 40% (>2000 ml)	HR > 140, ↓ BP, RR > 35, confused/lethargic, urine output - negligible, capillary refill > 3-4 sec.

Management of Adults with Blunt Abdominal Trauma

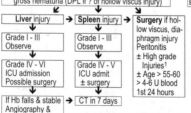

Begin Resuscitation - Immediate Bedside Ultrasound
⬇

Stable Vitals
CT if abdominal pain, distracting injury, altered LOC, gross hematuria (DPL if ? of hollow viscus injury)

Unstable Vitals
DPL 1st unless US shows hemoperitoneum

Liver injury → **Spleen** injury → **Surgery** if hollow viscus, diaphragm injury, Peritonitis ± High grade Injuries[1] ± Age > 55-60 > 4-6 U blood 1st 24 hours

Immediate Surgery
Refractory Low BP
Peritoneal signs
Diaphragm injury
Pneumoperitoneum
Positive DPL
Cannot assess mental status (controversial)

Grade I - III Observe → Grade I - III Observe

Grade IV - VI ICU admission Possible surgery → Grade IV - V ICU admit ± surgery

If Hb falls & stable Angiography & Embolization → CT in 7 days

→ No success → Surgery

Surg Clin North Am 1996; 76: 763.
J Trauma 1998;44:283.

Diagnostic Evaluation of Suspected Renal Trauma
Mechanism and Clinical Features

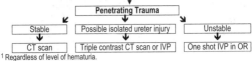

Blunt trauma[1] with pelvic or abdomen trauma, ↓ BP or gross hematuria	Blunt trauma with minor mechanism, normal BP and no gross hematuria
CT scan of abdomen/pelvis, consider surgery if avulsion, main vessel injury, or shattered kidney	Follow-up urinalysis alone, consider CT or IVP if persistent or worsening hematuria

Penetrating Trauma

Stable	Possible isolated ureter injury	Unstable
CT scan	Triple contrast CT scan or IVP	One shot IVP in OR

[1] Regardless of level of hematuria.
[2] Use triple contrast (IV, oral, rectal).   *Emerg Med Clin North Am* 1998; 16: 145.

Diagnostic Adjuncts in Blunt Abdominal Trauma

Physical examination: 20% with left lower rib fractures have injured spleen and 10% with right lower rib fractures have injured liver. Nonspecific indicators of liver damage include AST or ALT ≥ 130 IU/L and laparotomy need = base deficit ≤ -6.

Diagnostic tests	Positive Diagnostic Peritoneal Lavage
(1) <u>Computed tomography</u> may miss hollow viscus, pancreatic, mesenteric, and diaphragm injury. It requires hemodynamically stability. Oral contrast only aids in detecting < 1% additional pathology on CT, increases aspiration + adds time. (*Ann Emerg Med* 1997; 30:7) (2) <u>Diagnostic peritoneal lavage</u> (DPL) is more sensitive than CT for identifying need for laparotomy> DPL has more	Aspiration of ≥ 10 ml of gross blood Blunt or penetrating trauma abdomen ≥ 100,000 RBC's/ml ≥ 20,000-100,000 RBC's/ml equivocal Penetrating trauma lower chest ≥ 5,000 RBC/ml White blood cells ≥ 500/ml (4h lag) Lavage amylase ≥ 20 IU/L Lavage alkaline phosphatase ≥ 3 IU/L Bile, food or vegetable matter

false positive results and leads to unnecessary laparotomy in many cases.
(3) <u>Ultrasound</u> is less sensitive than DPL in detecting peritoneal blood (80-90% vs 98% for DPL), although US detects hemoperitoneum in most that require surgery.

Penetrating Abdominal Trauma

Indications for Laparotomy	
• Unstable vital signs	• Bowel protrusion or evisceration
• Peritoneal signs	• Impaled or embedded weapon
• Evidence of diaphragm injury	• Gun shot wound to abdomen[1]
• Significant GI bleeding	• Positive DPL (see above)

[1]Debate exists as to need for laparotomy in stab wound entering peritoneum.

Penetrating Flank or Back Injuries - Management

- Immediate celiotomy if shock, or obvious intraperitoneal or vascular injury.
- CT scan with triple contrast (oral, IV, and rectal) if no signs or symptoms of significant injury or gross hematuria alone in a hemodynamically stable patient.
- Angiography consider if significant retroperitoneal hematoma/bleeding

---

Trauma - Chest Injuries

Myocardial Contusion

Overview & ED Diagnosis	Features of Myocardial Contusion
The most common injuries are to (1) RV(2) anterior septum, & (3) anterior apical LV <u>Diagnosis</u>: CXR, ECG, & O₂ sat. CXR: pulmonary contusion, 1st or 2nd rib fractures, clavicle or sternal fractures, CHF. ECG findings may take 24 h to develop. Cardiac markers are not useful diagnostically.	Anginal pain (1-3 d after trauma) unrelieved by nitroglycerin External thoracic trauma (73%) Tachycardia (70%) Friction rub Beck's triad (cardiac tamponade) ↓BP, JVD, ↑HR (present in < 50%)

Radiologic Studies	ECG in Myocardial Contusion	
(1) Echo - RV wall dyskinesia ± chamber dilation. Echo identifies most problems that require treatment.	Sinus tachycardia	70%
	Nonspecific ST-T changes	60%
(2) Radionuclide angiography - assesses ejection fraction (EF). LVEF < 50% or RVEF < 40% are abnormal.	Repolarization disturbances	61%
	Atrial arrhythmias or	
	conduction defects	12%
(3) Single Photon Emission CT (SPECT) – can detect contusions/ischemia.	Ventricular dysrhythmias	22%
	Normal ECG	12%
	Myocardial infarction	2%

Management
Consider admission for monitoring if ECG changes, cardiac disease, co-existing trauma or > 45-55 years. Consider Echo or other test (2-3 above). Additional studies are only performed if problems/complications. (e.g. arrhythmia, hemodynamic instability). If < 45 years old, normal ECG & tachycardia resolves, discharge after 4 h observation/cardiac monitoring.

Traumatic Thoracic Aortic Rupture

Only 10-20% of patients survive to reach the ED. Rupture most frequently occurs at the fixed immobile ligamentum arteriosum due to a rapid deceleration injury.

Clinical Features	CXR in Thoracic Aortic Rupture
• Retrosternal or intra-scapular pain	• ↑ mediastinal width[1] (52-90%)
• Dyspnea, stridor, hoarse, dysphagia	• Obscured aortic knob
• ↑ or ↓BP (mean BP 152/98)	• Opacified aorticopulmonary window
• Depressed lower extremity BP	• NG rube > 2 cm to the right of T4
• Systolic intrascapular/precordial murmur, swelling at base of neck	• Tracheal stripe > 5 mm from right lung
• Sternal, scapula or multiple rib fractures (esp. 1st or 2nd rib	• Left main stem bronchus 40° below horizontal
• Chest tube with initial output > 750 ml	• Left hemothorax/apical pleural cap
	• NORMAL CXR (up to 15%)

1 MW on erect PA CXR > 6 cm, on supine AP > 8 cm , > 7.5 at aortic knob or MW at aortic knob/chest width > 0.25 all correlate with thoracic aortic rupture.

Diagnosis of Thoracic Aortic Rupture

- Spiral CT scan - > 97-100% sensitive for aortic rupture.
- Transesophageal echo- very accurate - best reserved for the unstable patient
- Intraarterial Digital Subtraction Angiography (IA-DSA) - 100% sensitive in 1 series

Management of Suspected Thoracic Aortic Rupture

- Perform resuscitation of ABC's as per resuscitation of all trauma patients.
- Some experts state that repair of life threatening hemoperitoneum and brain stem herniation are the major disorders that take precedence over aortic rupture
- Maintain systolic BP ≤ 120 mm Hg by 1st controlling fluids, sedation, and pain. Consider short acting IV agents β-blockade (esmolol + *Nipride*). See page 207.
- Contact thoracic surgeon and prepare for surgery.

Genitourinary Trauma

Urethral Trauma

Overview	Retrograde Urethrogram Indications[1]
Pelvic fractures cause most proximal injuries while anterior injuries are usually due to falls, or straddle. Perform abdominal, perineal, & rectal exam, and obtain urethrogram if injury suspected	Penile, scrotal, perineal trauma Blood at urethral meatus High riding prostate on examination Suspected pelvis fracture (*controversial*) Inability to easily pass Foley catheter
Management	*Retrograde Urethrogram Technique[1]*
If a partial urethral disruption, a urologist may attempt to gently pass a 14-16 F catheter. If unsuccessful or a complete urethral disruption is found, a supra-pubic catheter will need to be placed.	Obtain preinjection KUB film Place Cooke adapter on 60 ml syringe. (Do not use Foley) Inject 10-15 ml of contrast in 60 seconds TAP/oblique xrays during last 10 sec

Bladder Trauma

Overview	Cystogram Indications
All with bladder trauma have pelvic fractures, abdominal trauma requiring CT, or gross hematuria (98%). If gross hematuria perform cystogram. Abdominal CT scan can miss this injury. CT abdomen before cystogram so dye does not obscure CT.	Penetrating injury to low abdomen/pelvis Blunt abdominal or perineal trauma with (1) gross hematuria, (2) blood at the urethral meatus, (3) pelvic fracture or (4) abnormal retrograde urethrogram or (5) inability to void or minimal urine from Foley catheter
Management	*Cystogram Technique*
Intraperitoneal rupture releases dye into abdomen,. Exploration of abdomen + repair often required. Extraperitoneal rupture is in perivesical tissues, while washout may show dye behind bladder. Treat with catheter (Foley if small, suprapubic if large) alone.	After urethrogram, insert Foley.Obtain baseline KUB, Instill dye[1] by gravity until 400 ml or bladder contraction Clamp Foley, Obtain (AP + oblique) Xrays, then empty bladder +/- wash out bladder with saline solution Then obtain final KUB with oblique film

[1]Use *Hypaque* 50%, *Cystografin* 40, or *Renografin* 60, or non-ionic dye (*Omnipaque* or *Isovue*) diluted to ≤ 10% solution with NS.

High Yield Criteria for Cranial CT in Trauma Patients with a GCS of 13-15

Major Risk Factors	Utility of Major Criteria in Predicting Need for Neurologic intervention[1]	
• Failure to reach GCS of 15 in 2h		
• Suspected open skull fracture	Sensitivity	100% (92-100%)
• Any sign of basal skull fracture	Specificity	68.7% (67-70%)
• Vomiting > 1 episode	Utility of Major + Minor Criteria in Predicting Clinically Important CNS Injury[2]	
• Age > 64 years		
Minor Risk Factors	Sensitivity	98.4% (96-99%)
• Amnesia before impact > 30 min	Specificity	49.6% (48-51%)
• Dangerous mechanism below (Pedestrian struck, assault by blunt object, fall > 3 feet/5 stairs, heavy object fall on head, vehicle ejection)	1. death ≤ 7 d, craniotomy, elevation of skull fracture, ICP monitor, intubate for head injury 2. any CT injury requiring admission and neurologic follow up	

Lancet 2001, 357: 1391-1396. Numbers in parentheses are 95% confidence intervals.

Management of Severe Head Injury (Glasgow Coma Scale ≤ 8)
General Trauma Evaluation (page 169)

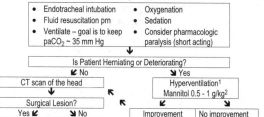

- • Endotracheal intubation
- • Fluid resuscitation prn
- • Ventilate – goal is to keep $paCO_2$ ~ 35 mm Hg

- • Oxygenation
- • Sedation
- • Consider pharmacologic paralysis (short acting)

Is Patient Herniating or Deteriorating?

↙ No   ↘ Yes

| CT scan of the head | | Hyperventilation[1] Mannitol 0.5 - 1 g/kg[2] |

Surgical Lesion?

Yes ↙   No ↘   Improvement   No improvement

| To Operating Room | ICU admit Monitor ICP Treat ICP |

To Operating Room

[1] Hyperventilation should only be instituted for brief periods if there is an acute neurologic deterioration. A $PaCO_2$ ≤ 35 mm Hg will ↓ cerebral perfusion & can worsen outcome.
[2] Mannitol is only indicated prior to ICP monitoring if signs of herniation or progressive neurologic deterioration occur. Bolus therapy is most effective. Keep serum Osm < 320.

Am Ass Neuro Surg & Brain Trauma Foundation 1996

Trauma - Neck Injuries - Penetrating

Wounds through platysma
muscle are of major concern.
(A) Some experts believe
that Zone I and III injuries
generally require angio-
graphy to identify major
vascular injury while Zone II
injuries generally do not.
(B) Others manage
penetrating injuries per the
algorithm outlined below.

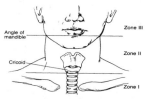

Used with permission. Tintinalli J et al. *Emergency Medicine.*
A comprehensive study guide. McGraw Hill. 1996; 1156. Figure 217-3

Initial Management of Patient with Penetrating Neck Injury	
Airway	• Expanding hematomas, stridor, or other indicators of impending airway compromise mandate endotracheal intubation.
Breathing	• Obtain CXR to exclude pneumothorax. Chest tube prn.
Circulation	• Control bleeding by direct compression and give NS or blood.
Other Evaluation	• Contact consultants early & exclude cervical, neuro., vascular, airway, lung,GI injury clinically, or via Xray, or exploration.

Management of the Neck Injury Based on Clinical Exam

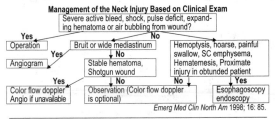

Emerg Med Clin North Am 1998; 16: 85.

Pelvis and Extremity Trauma

Criteria for Pelvis Radiography Following Blunt Trauma

- Glasgow coma scale < 14
- Intoxication with drugs or alcohol
- Hypotension or gross hematuria
- Lower extremity neurologic deficit
- Femur fracture or painful/tender pelvis, symphysis pubis, or iliac spine

- Pain, swelling, bruise to medial thigh, groin genitalia, suprapubic area, back
- Instability of pelvis to anterior-posterior or lateral-medial pressure
- Pain with abduction, adduction, rotation, or flexion of either hip

Criteria – 100% sensitive. *Ann Emerg Med* 1988; 17: 488; and *J Trauma* 1993; 34: 236.

Initial Management of Pelvic Fractures (*EM Clin North Am* 2000;18:1)

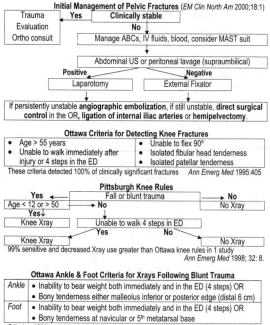

Trauma Evaluation Ortho consult → **Yes** | **Clinically stable**

No ↓

Manage ABCs, IV fluids, blood, consider MAST suit

Abdominal US or peritoneal lavage (supraumbilical)

Positive → Laparotomy   **Negative** → External Fixator

If persistently unstable **angiographic embolization**, if still unstable, **direct surgical control** in the OR, **ligation of internal iliac arteries** or **hemipelvectomy**.

Ottawa Criteria for Detecting Knee Fractures

- Age > 55 years
- Unable to walk immediately after injury or 4 steps in the ED
- Unable to flex 90º
- Isolated fibular head tenderness
- Isolated patellar tenderness

These criteria detected 100% of clinically significant fractures   *Ann Emerg Med* 1995:405

Pittsburgh Knee Rules

Yes ← Fall or blunt trauma → **No**

Age < 12 or > 50 → **No** | **No Xray**

Yes ↓

Knee Xray | Unable to walk 4 steps in ED

Yes → Knee Xray   **No** → No Xray

99% sensitive and decreased Xray use greater than Ottawa knee rules in 1 study
Ann Emerg Med 1998; 32: 8.

Ottawa Ankle & Foot Criteria for Xrays Following Blunt Trauma

Ankle	• Inability to bear weight both immediately and in the ED (4 steps) OR
	• Bony tenderness either malleolus inferior or posterior edge (distal 6 cm)
Foot	• Inability to bear weight both immediately and in the ED (4 steps) OR
	• Bony tenderness at navicular or 5th metatarsal base

Criteria - 100% sensitive in detecting clinically significant ankle/foot fractures.
Ann Emerg Med 1992; 21: 384-390.

Cervical, Thoracic, Lumbar Spine, Shoulder Injuries

NEXUS Cervical Spine Xray Criteria[1]

• Neck tenderness - midline	• Intoxication with drugs or alcohol
• Motor or sensory deficit	• Distracting painful injury
• Altered mental status	

[1] These criteria were 99% sensitive, with a 99.9% negative predictive value (*if features absent 0.1% probability of fracture*) in detecting clinically significant C spine fractures.
N Engl J Med 2000; 343: 94.

Canadian C-Spine Rule (CCR)

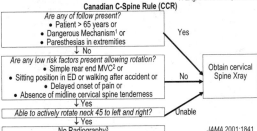

Are any of follow present?
- Patient > 65 years or
- Dangerous Mechanism[1] or
- Paresthesias in extremities
↓ No — Yes

Are any low risk factors present allowing rotation?
- Simple rear end MVC[2] or
- Sitting position in ED or walking after accident or
- Delayed onset of pain or
- Absence of midline cervical spine tenderness
↓ Yes — No

Able to actively rotate neck 45 to left and right? — Unable
↓ Yes

No Radiography[3] → Obtain cervical Spine Xray

JAMA 2001;1841

[1] Fall ≥ 3 feet/5 stairs, axial load to head (e.g. diving), high speed MVC (>100 kilometers(65 miles)/hour), rollover, ejection, motorized recreational vehicles, bicycle crash
[2] Pushed into oncoming traffic, hit by bus/truck, rollover, hit at high speed.
[3] These criteria are 100% sensitive (98-100%, 95% Confidence interval) in detecting clinically important C-spine fractures. A prospective study found the CCR to be more sensitive than NEXUS rule for identifying C-spine injuries in stable alert patients in Canada. *N Engl J Med* 2003; 349: 2510; *JAMA* 2001; 286: 1841

Indications for Thoracolumbar Spine Radiographs in Blunt Trauma

Back pain or tenderness	Ejection from motorcycle/vehicle
Neurologic deficit	Motor vehicle crash ≥ 50 miles per hour
Glasgow Coma Scale ≤ 14	Major distracting injury
Drug or alcohol Intoxication	• pelvic or long bone fracture
Fall ≥ 10 feet	• intrathoracic or abdominal injury

Criteria were 100% sensitive in detecting thoracolumbar fractures in all 5 studies cited. Mechanism (fall, MCV, ejection) did not add to 100% sensitivity in several studies.
J Emerg Med 2003; 1; *Am J Surg* 1995;681, *J Trauma* 1993 85; 1994;673; 1995;1110

High-Yield Criteria for Shoulder Xrays in the Emergency Department

• Shoulder deformity or swelling	• History of fall (with age ≥ 43.5 years)
• Abnormal range of motion	*AJEM* 1998;560; *J Rheumatol* 2000; 200

These criteria were 100% sensitive in detecting clinically significant abnormal Xrays (fracture, 3rd AC joint, infection, cancer) in 2 studies.

Spinal Cord Injury Syndromes[1]

Anterior Cord Syndrome	Central Cord Syndrome
• Flexion or vertical compression injury to anterior cord or spinal artery • Complete motor paralysis • Hyperalgesia with preserved touch and proprioception (position sense) • Loss of pain and temperature sense • Most likely cord injury to require surgery	• Hyperextension injury • Motor weakness in hands > arms • Legs are unaffected or less affected • Variable bladder/sensory dysfunction • Prognosis is generally good and most do not require surgery

	Brown-Sequard Syndrome
Complete Cord Injury	• Hemisection of cord • Ipsilateral weakness • Ipsilateral loss of proprioception • Lose contralateral pain/temperature
• Flaccid below injury level • Warm skin ,↓BP,↓HR • Sensation may be preserved • ↓ Sympathetics ± priapism • Absent deep tendon reflexes • If lasts > 24 h will be permanent	**Posterior Cord Syndrome**
	• Pain, tingling, of neck and hands • 1/3 have upper extremity weakness • Mild form of central cord syndrome

[1] see page 114 for dermatomes, muscles, and reflexes.

Steroid Protocol for Treatment of Acute Spinal Cord Injury

Indications	• Acute spinal cord injury presenting within **8 hours** of injury.
Contra-indications	• Age < 13 y (*controversial*) • Isolated nerve root injury • Cauda equina syndrome • Penetrating cord trauma • Life-threatening illness/injury independent of spinal cord injury • Patients who were pregnant or on steroids were excluded from original study and may be relative contraindications
Protocol	• Methylprednisolone (*Solu-Medrol*) 30 mg/kg IV over 15 minutes, then wait 45 minutes • If < 3 hours since injury, *Solu-Medrol* 5.4 mg/kg/h over 23 hours • If 3-8 hours since injury, *Solu-Medrol* 5.4 mg/kg/h over 47 hours

New Engl J Med 1990; 322: 1405 & *JAMA* 1997; 277: 1597.

Urologic Disorders

The Painful Scrotum

Feature	Torsion of Testicle	Epididymitis & Orchitis	Torsion of Testicular Appendix
Frequency, age 0-20 yr	25-50%	10-25%	30-50%
Frequency, age 20-29	20%	80%	0%
Pain onset	acute onset	gradual onset	gradual onset
Pain location	testis, groin, or abdomen	testes, groin, epididymis	testis or upper pole
Prior similar episodes	often	occasional	rare
Fever	rare	up to 1/3	rare
Dysuria	rare	common	rare
Testicle/Scrotum	horizontal high riding testis	firm, red, warm epididymis or testis (>70%)	usually nontender, blue-dot upper testis
Cremasteric reflex	usually absent	may be present	may be present
Pyuria	up to 10%	25-60%	rare
Doppler/Nuclear scan	↓ flow	↑flow	normal flow

Accuracy of Diagnostic Tests for Testicular Torsion in Adults	Test	Sensitivity	Specificity
	Doppler ultrasound	80-90%	80-90%
	Color Doppler US	86-100%	100%
	Nuclear scan	80-90%	>95%

Urology Clin North Am 1996; Radiology Clin North Am 1997;

Management of Suspected Testicular Torsion

- In men under 40 with a painful testicle, assume torsion until proven otherwise.
- Contact a urologist immediately, as early surgical detorsion has the best chance of saving the testicle.
- If the clinical suspicion is low to moderate, consider diagnostic test above after consultation with urologist.
- An attempt to manually detorse the testicle may restore blood flow. To manually detorse, rotate the anterior aspect of the testicle towards the ipsilateral thigh (like opening a book). The testicle will need to be torsed at least 360 degrees. If successful, the patient will experience a marked relief of pain, and the testicle will develop a normal lie (position in scrotum).

Select Emergency Drugs & Infusions

ALLERGY	diphenhydramine (*Benadryl*): 50 mg IV/IM. epinephrine: 0.1-0.5 mg SC (1:1000 solution), may repeat after 20 minutes. methylprednisolone (*Solu-Medrol*): 125 mg IV/IM.
HYPERTENSION	enalapril (*Vasotec*): 1.25-5 mg IV over 5 minutes esmolol (*Brevibloc*): 500 mcg/kg IV over 1 min, then titrate 50-300mcg/kg/min fenoldopam (*Corlopam*): Start 0.1 mcg/kg/min, titrate up to 1.6 mcg/kg/mn labetalol (*Normodyne*): 0.25 mg/kg IV, may double dose q 10-15 min prn (maximum cumulative total dose of 300 mg or 2 mg/kg – whichever is less) nitroglycerin (*Tridil*): Start 10-20 mcg/min IV, titrate up to 100 mcg/min sodium nitroprusside (*Nipride*): 0.3-10 mcg/kg/minute
DYSRHYTHMIAS / CARDIAC ARREST	adenosine (*Adenocard*): SVT (not A-fib/flutter): 6 mg rapid IV & flush, preferably through a central line or proximal IV. If no response after 1-2 minutes then 12 mg. A third dose of 12 mg may be given prn. amiodarone (*Cordarone, Pacerone*): Life-threatening ventricular arrhythmia: Load 150 mg IV over 10 min, then 1 mg/min x 6h, then 0.5 mg/min x 18h. atropine: 0.5-1.0 mg IV or 2-3 mg (in 10 ml) via ET diltiazem (*Cardizem*): Rapid atrial fib: bolus 0.25 mg/kg or 20 mg IV over 2 min. May repeat 0.35 mg/kg or 25 mg IV 15 min later. Infuse 5-15 mg/h. epinephrine: 1 mg IV (2-2.5 mg in 10 ml ET) for cardiac arrest. [1:10,000] lidocaine (*Xylocaine*): 1 mg/kg IV, then 0.5 mg/kg q5-10min prn to max 3 mg/kg. Maintenance 2g in 250ml D5W (8 mg/ml) at 1-4 mg/min (7-30 ml/h) vasopressin (*Pitressin*, ADH): Ventricular fibrillation: 40 units IV once. May also be effective in asystolic cardiac arrest.
PRESSORS	dobutamine: 250 mg in 250ml D5W (1 mg/ml) at 2.5-20 mcg/kg/min dopamine: 400 mg in 250ml D5W (1600 mcg/ml) at 2-20 mcg/kg/min. Doses in mcg/kg/min: 2-5 = dopaminergic, 5-10 = beta, >10 = alpha. norepinephrine (*Levophed*): 4 mg in 500 ml D5W (8 mcg/ml) at 0.5-10 mcg/min. (max 30 mcg/min) phenylephrine (*Neo-Synephrine*): 100-500 mcg boluses IV. Infusion for hypotension: 20 mg in 250ml D5W (80 mcg/ml), start at 100-180 mcg/min (75-135 ml/h). Once BP stable, decrease to maintenance of 40-60 mcg/min
INTUBATION	etomidate (*Amidate*): 0.3-0.4 mg/kg IV. methohexital (*Brevital*): 1-1.5 mg/kg IV. rocuronium (*Zemuron*): 0.6-1.2 mg/kg IV. succinylcholine (*Anectine*): 1-1.5 mg/kg IV. thiopental (*Pentothal*): 3-5 mg/kg IV.
SEIZURES	diazepam (*Valium*): 2-20 mg IV, or 0.2-0.5 mg/kg rectal gel up to 20 mg PR fosphenytoin (*Cerebyx*): Load 15-20 phenytoin equivalents per kg either IM or IV no faster than 100-150 mg/min lorazepam (*Ativan*): 0.1 mg/kg up to 3-4 mg IV/IM phenobarbital: 200-320 mg IV at 60 mg/min, status epilepticus give 20 mg/kg phenytoin (*Dilantin*): 20 mg/kg up to 1000 mg IV no faster than 50 mg/min

GLOBE FEARON
Pearson Learning Group